Dementia Care
A Practical Approach

Dementia Care
A Practical Approach

Edited by

Grahame Smith
Liverpool John Moores University, UK

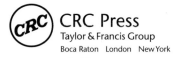

CRC Press
Taylor & Francis Group
Boca Raton   London   New York

CRC Press is an imprint of the
Taylor & Francis Group, an **informa** business

CRC Press
Taylor & Francis Group
6000 Broken Sound Parkway NW, Suite 300
Boca Raton, FL 33487-2742

© 2016 by Taylor & Francis Group, LLC
CRC Press is an imprint of Taylor & Francis Group, an Informa business

No claim to original U.S. Government works

Printed and bound in India by Replika Press Pvt. Ltd.

Printed on acid-free paper
Version Date: 20151119

International Standard Book Number-13: 978-1-4822-4573-8 (Paperback)

Library of Congress Cataloging-in-Publication Data

Names: Smith, Grahame, editor.
Title: Dementia care : a practical approach / editor, Grahame Michael Smith.
Other titles: Dementia care (Smith)
Description: Boca Raton, FL : CRC Press, 2016. | Includes bibliographical references and index. | Description based on
    print version record and CIP data provided by publisher; resource not viewed.
Identifiers: LCCN 2015045102 (print) | LCCN 2015044026 (ebook) | ISBN 9781482245745 (e-book) | ISBN
    9781482245752 (e-book - VITAL BOOK) | ISBN 9781482245769 (ePUB) | ISBN 9781482245738 (paperback : alk.
    paper)
Subjects: | MESH: Dementia--therapy--Great Britain. | Patient Care--methods--Great Britain.
Classification: LCC RC521 (print) | LCC RC521 (ebook) | NLM WM 220 | DDC 362.1968/300941--dc23
LC record available at http://lccn.loc.gov/2015045102

Visit the Taylor & Francis Web site at
http://www.taylorandfrancis.com

and the CRC Press Web site at
http://www.crcpress.com

Contents

Welcome

I hope you will find this book useful in your lifelong learning journey, whether it is as a practitioner, a person with dementia, an informal caregiver, or someone who just wants to know more about the subject. It is an academic text, and it has been written with the trainee health care and social care practitioner in mind; in terms of writing style, it is intended to be open, accessible and pragmatic. "… the function of inquiry is not to represent reality, but rather to enable us to act more effectively" (Edward, 2000: 705).

Dementia is a personal and a societal challenge. The role of the health and social care practitioner is to meet this challenge with hope and compassion, to be the change you wish to see in the world (attributed to Mahatma Gandhi).

Ultimately, success will be measured by the people the practitioner works for, people living with dementia; their feedback will enable the practitioner to improve his or her practice for the betterment of all.

THE CHALLENGE

It is estimated that there are 835,000 people with dementia in the United Kingdom and that most people living with dementia live in their own home, with a sizeable proportion living alone (Alzheimer's Society, 2014). There are estimated to be 40,000 younger people (i.e. under the age of 65 years) with dementia living in the United Kingdom. These figures may be an underestimation of the true figures due to the difficulties people experience in receiving a diagnosis of dementia (Alzheimer's Society, 2014). As people live longer, it is predicted that the incidence of dementia will double by 2030, and by 2050 more than triple (Woods et al., 2013; World Health Organisation [WHO], 2012). The challenge for society—locally, nationally and internationally—is ensuring that care provision both now and in the future is fit for purpose; it must also have an emphasis on continually improving the quality of life and well-being of those living with dementia (WHO, 2012; European Commission, 2009).

On a personal level, living with dementia can be challenging and sometimes overwhelming; where the right support is in place, then living well with dementia can become a reality rather than just a societal aspiration (Alzheimer's Society, 2014). To achieve this aspiration, it has to be recognised that there is more to be done, especially in the following areas (Alzheimer's Society, 2014):

- Diagnosis
- Health and social care provision
- Quality of care
- Dementia-friendly communities
- Research

Health care and social care practitioners who work with people living with dementia, whether in a specialist dementia role or not, will play a crucial role in the delivery of the means to realize this societal aspiration. This may be at an operational level or a strategic level:

Dementia is now a public and political priority in a way that it has never been before. Starting with England in 2009 and followed by Wales and Northern Ireland in 2011, national plans on dementia were launched in each country increasing the political attention across the nations. In England, the strategy on dementia was supported by the Prime Minister's challenge on dementia, which promised 'to push further and faster on major improvements in care and research by 2015' (Department of Health [DH], 2012). (Alzheimer's Society, 2014: 3)

This strategic commitment to improve dementia care delivery is underpinned by the necessity to promote care that is person centred, holistic, and compassionate (Kitwood, 1997; Mast, 2014; Francis, 2013). Most practitioners would argue that they deliver compassionate care; however, after a number of high-profile incidents, there is a concerted effort to ensure that compassion is a value that is systematically embedded within the culture of health and social care:

The reports on Winterbourne View and Mid Staffordshire will be a call to action for everyone, Government, the NHS Commissioning Board, the NMC [Nursing and Midwifery Council], the Care Quality Commission, the trades unions and all the other players in the system, to get behind staff and support them in their professional instincts for compassion. (Commissioning Board, 2012: 12)

It is important to recognise that dementia is everybody's business; the global population is 'aging', and the potential increase in the prevalence of dementia is a significant socioeconomic challenge to society as a whole (Woods et al., 2013; WHO, 2012). Globally,

… the total estimated worldwide costs of dementia were US$ 604 billion in 2010. (WHO, 2012: 2)

And in the United Kingdom,

With an aging population the numbers of people with dementia in the UK are increasing and so are the costs. Dementia now costs the UK economy £26 billion a year, with this price tag set to rise. (Alzheimer's Society, 2014: 1)

This means that practitioners not only have to be compassionate, paying careful attention to improving the quality of life of people living with dementia, but also will have to consider new ways of working that manage costs (Woods et al., 2013; Ham, Dixon, & Brooke, 2012). One way of doing this is to develop innovative ways of working, which may include the use of assistive technologies; the viability of this approach is dependent on practitioners sharing examples of good practice (Woods et al., 2013; Alzheimer Cooperative Valuation in Europe [ALCOVE], 2012; European Commission, 2010; Dewsbury & Linskell, 2011). Innovative solutions will only be sustainable in the long term where they fit the real needs of people living with dementia; this includes solutions that are designed to support people who have just been diagnosed through to solutions that support people at the end of life (Woods, 2004; Prince, Bryce, & Ferri, 2011).

Taking this into consideration, it is fundamental that the innovation process places people living with dementia at the heart of the process in a way that is person centred and values them as equal partners (Kitwood, 1997; Richardson & Cotton, 2011; DH, 2011; Weber, 2011).

Health and social care practitioners will work with people living with dementia in a variety of settings and in diverse roles. They may not see themselves as specialists in the field of dementia although it is incumbent on them to have a good level of dementia awareness (DH, 2009). Not all people exhibiting the signs and symptoms of dementia have been diagnosed, and on this basis, they may not have been receiving the level of support that is required (Alzheimer's Society, 2014). Barriers to receiving a timely diagnosis still exist; these include the following:

lack of strategic approach to dementia at local level; low public awareness of dementia; poor understanding of dementia by health and social care professionals; disinclination to diagnose in areas where support services are not available; and limited partnership between health and social care providers. (APPG [All-Party Parliamentary Group on Dementia], 2012). (Alzheimer's Society, 2014: 9)

Assisting people to overcome these barriers is a key part of the practitioner's role; once a diagnosis is assigned, the practitioner will also need to be skilled in delivering good quality care. Interventions no longer concentrate just on symptom control; they should be holistic, considering the whole of the person, including the person's existing social networks (DH, 2009; Kitwood, 1997). Living well with dementia is the overarching goal and is one that this book shares along with adopting a 'strengths approach' to the delivery of care.

LEARNING THAT INFORMS PRACTICE

Living well with dementia is a multifaceted notion, the DH (2009) describes living well with dementia as a three part process:

encourage help-seeking and help-offering (referral for diagnosis) by changing public and professional attitudes, understanding and behaviour;
    make early diagnosis and treatment the rule rather than the exception; and achieve this by locating the responsibility for the diagnosis of mild and moderate dementia in a specifically commissioned part of the system that can, first, make the diagnoses well, second, break those diagnoses sensitively and well to those affected, and third, provide individuals with immediate treatment, care and peer and professional support as needed; and
    enable people with dementia and their carers to live well with dementia by the provision of good quality care for all with dementia from diagnosis to the end of life, in the community, in hospitals and in care homes. (DH, 2009: 21)

Before considering the specific skills a health and social care practitioner needs to possess, it is important to acknowledge that pre-qualifying programmes that are professionally accredited by the Nursing and Midwifery Council (NMC) or Health and Care Professions Council (HCPC), depending on the programme, will provide a good generic background on which to develop specific dementia-related skills. As an example, the NMC's (2010) Standards for Pre-registration Nursing Education aim to

… enable nurses to give and support high quality care in rapidly changing environments. They reflect how future services are likely to be delivered, acknowledge future public health priorities and address the challenges of long-term conditions, an ageing population, and providing more care outside hospitals. Nurses must be equipped to lead, delegate, supervise and challenge other nurses and healthcare professionals. They must be able to develop practice, and promote and sustain change. As graduates they must be able to think analytically, use problem-solving approaches and evidence in decision-making, keep up with technical advances and meet future expectations. (Nursing & Midwifery Council, 2010: 4–5)

Irrespective of the nurse's field of practice (adult, children, learning disabilities, or mental health), there is the expectation that the nurse at the point of registration will have the generic skills and knowledge to provide good-quality dementia care (NMC, 2010). In terms of specific skills and knowledge,

The need to develop an effective and informed workforce in dementia has received significant attention over the last few years within national dementia strategies and plans. In order to achieve good quality dementia care it is essential that all health and social care staff have the necessary skills to provide the best quality of care in the roles and settings where they work. (Higher Education for Dementia Network [HEDN], 2013: 3)

In recent years, there has been a drive to improve the care of people living with dementia by providing dementia awareness training:

All NHS staff that look after people with dementia will go through a dementia awareness programme (Tier 1 foundation level dementia training). (DH, 2014: 16)

Tier 1 foundation training level learning outcomes have been identified as the following:

- Better diagnosis, treatment and care of those with dementia;
- Staff will have greater awareness and confidence to support patients affected by dementia;
- Staff will be able to identify the early symptoms of dementia;
- Staff will be aware of the needs of patients affected by dementia and their families and carers to enable them to provide safe, dignified and compassionate care;
- GPs [general practitioners] will be able to identify and work with patients affected by dementia;
- Staff will be able to signpost patients and carers to appropriate support;
- Staff will have raised awareness of the increased likelihood of mental health problems presenting in those with Long Term Conditions. (NHS, Health Education South West)

The HEDN (2013) provides a framework that is consistent with these tier 1 outcomes; it also is more extensive in scope in that it is 'intended to guide the content of higher education pro-grammes developed for health and social care professionals' (HEDN, 2013: 3). The following list is a summary of the content areas (HEDN, 2013):

- Identification and assessment of dementia
- Understanding the experience of and communicating with people with dementia
- Creating effective partnerships with carers and families

- Equality, diversity and inclusion in dementia care
- Supporting people in the early stages of dementia
- Developing person-centred care, assessment and care planning
- Holistic health for people with dementia
- Supporting the daily life of people with dementia
- Pharmacology relating to the needs of people with dementia
- Psychosocial approaches for people with dementia
- Key professional abilities and collaborative working
- Understanding legal aspects of working with people with dementia
- Understanding ethical issues in caring for people with dementia
- End-of-life palliative care
- Environment
- Research, policy and service development in dementia care

Both the tier 1 learning outcomes and the HEDN (2013) curriculum for UK dementia education underpin the structure and the content of this book.

BOOK STRUCTURE

There are times when people with dementia can exhibit 'risky' behaviours, and health and social care practitioners will be required to manage those risks in a way that is enabling:

Risk enablement is based on the idea that the process of measuring risk involves balancing the positive benefits from taking risks against the negative effects of attempting to avoid risk altogether. For example, the risk of getting lost if a person with dementia goes out unaccompanied needs to be set against the possible risks of boredom and frustration from remaining inside. (DH, 2010: 8)

Taking a risk enablement approach is compatible with a 'strengths approach':

Risk enablement recognises the strengths that each person with dementia possesses and builds on the abilities that he or she has retained. (DH, 2010: 8)

In turn, a strengths-based approach or perspective

… strives to lead with the positive and values trust, respect, intentionality, and optimism. (Hirst, Lane, & Stares, 2013: 331)

Taking this into consideration, the intention of this book is to be optimistic and focus on how practitioners can enable people living with dementia to live well (DH, 2009). To do this, it is essential that the practitioner is person centred, compassionate, and partnership focused (Francis, 2013; DH, 2010). To support practitioners in their journey to enable people to live well with dementia, this book has been written and structured so that a strengths-based perspective is the theme. The content is underpinned by relevant policies and strategies, explicitly links to the relevant research evidence, and always values the voices of people living with dementia.

This book is primarily aimed at preregistration nursing students, but some aspects will also be useful to other health-care students in prequalifying education programmes. To ensure that

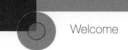

the book is a robust resource for students who are training to be health care and social care professionals the content has been mapped to the HCPC's and NMC's pre-qualifying requirements, the tier 1 dementia outcomes, and the curriculum for dementia education.

Every chapter has a core structure, aim(s) and objectives, core content, chapter summary, and reflection on learning. A scenario-based approach is used throughout to encourage the reader to consider how their learning can inform personal practice (Arnold & Thompson, 2009). It is acknowledged that the reader in a pre-qualifying programme will be constantly testing their experiences in this programme against the content of the book—this is actively encouraged as it is part of being a critical thinker (Smith, 2012). The reader may similarly not agree with some of the content or some of the points made, and if so, the reader is encouraged to undertake further research to support their position (Smith, 2012).

As noted, each chapter takes a common approach. Chapter 7, 'Living with Dementia', has a slightly different approach as it is based on the pure narrative experiences of people living with dementia. Chapter 14, 'Research', instead of using a scenario based on a practice experience, uses research exemplars. The authors of each chapter have extensive practice experience, whether as practitioners and/or people living with dementia, and therefore each chapter stands on its own merits.

REFERENCES

All-Party Parliamentary Group on Dementia. 2012. *Unlocking diagnosis*. London: Alzheimer's Society.

Alzheimer Cooperative Valuation in Europe. 2012. http://www.alcove-project.eu/index.php?option=com_content&view=article&id=45.

Alzheimer's Society. 2014. *Dementia 2014: Opportunity for Change.* London: Alzheimer's Society.

Arnold, L., & Thompson, K. 2009. Learning to learn through real world inquiry in the virtual paradigm. *Journal of Learning & Teaching Research*, 1: 6–33.

Commissioning Board: Chief Nursing Officer and DH Chief Nursing Adviser. 2012. *Compassion in Practice*. London: Department of Health and the NHS Commissioning Board.

Department of Health. 2009. *Living Well with Dementia: A National Dementia Strategy*. London: Department of Health.

Department of Health. 2010. *Nothing Ventured, Nothing Gained: Risk Guidance for People with Dementia*. London: Department of Health.

Department of Health. 2011. *NHS Operating Framework 2012–13*. London: Department of Health.

Department of Health. 2012. *Prime Minister's Challenge on Dementia: Delivering Major Improvements in Dementia Care and Research by 2015*. London: Department of Health.

Department of Health. 2014. *Delivering High Quality, Effective, Compassionate Care: Developing the Right People with the Right Skills and the Right Values—A Mandate from the Government to Health Education England: April 2014 to March 2015*. London: Department of Health.

Dewsbury, G., & Linskell, J. 2011. Smart home technology for safety and functional independence: The UK experience. *NeuroRehabilitation*, 28(3): 249–260.

Edward, C. (Ed.). 2000. *Concise Routledge Encyclopaedia of Philosophy*. London: Routledge.

European Commission. 2009. *Communication from the Commission to the European Parliament and the Council: On a European Initiative on Alzheimer's Disease and Other Dementias*. Brussels: European Commission.

European Commission. 2010. *INTERREG IVB: North West Europe 2007–2013*. Lille, France: INTERREG IVB.

Francis, R. 2013. *Report of the Mid Staffordshire NHS Foundation Trust Public Inquiry—Executive Summary*. London: Stationery Office.

Ham, C., Dixon, A., & Brooke, B. 2012. *Transforming the Delivery of Health and Social Care*. London: Kings Fund.

Higher Education for Dementia Network. 2013. *A Curriculum for UK Dementia Education*. London: Dementia UK.

Hirst, S.P., Lane, A., & Stares, R. 2013. Health promotion with older adults experiencing mental health challenges: A literature review of strength-based approaches. *Clinical Gerontologist*, 36(4): 329–355.

Kitwood, T. 1997. *Dementia Reconsidered*. London: Open University Press.

Mast, B. 2014. Whole person assessment and care planning. In *Excellence in Dementia Care*, 2nd edition, edited by Downs, M., & Bowers, B., 290–302. Maidenhead, England: Open University Press.

NHS, Health Education South West. Dementia Training Tier 1 Learning Outcomes. http://southwest.hee.nhs.uk/ourwork/dementia/tier1outcomes/ (accessed February 19, 2015).

Nursing and Midwifery Council. 2010. *Standards for Pre-registration Nursing Education*. London: Nursing and Midwifery Council.

Prince, M., Bryce, R., & Ferri, C. 2011. *World Alzheimer Report: The Benefits of Early Diagnosis and Intervention*. London: Alzheimer's Disease International.

Richardson, A., & Cotton, R. 2011. *No Health without Mental Health: Developing an Outcomes Based Approach*. London: NHS Confederation.

Smith, G. 2012. An introduction to psychological interventions. In *Psychological Interventions in Mental Health Nursing*, edited by Smith, G., 1–10. Maidenhead, England: Open University Press.

Weber, M.E.A. 2011. *Customer Co-creation in Innovations: A Protocol for Innovating with End Users*. Eindhoven, the Netherlands: Eindhoven University of Technology.

Woods, B. 2004. Invited commentary: Nonpharmacological interventions in dementia. *Advances in Psychiatric Treatments*, 10(3): 178–179.

Woods, L., Smith, G., Pendleton, J., & Parker, D. 2013. *Innovate Dementia Baseline Report: Shaping the Future for People Living with Dementia*. Liverpool, England: Liverpool John Moores University.

World Health Organisation. 2012. *Dementia: A Public Health Priority*. Geneva: World Health Organisation.

Contributors

Susan Ashton
Faculty of Education, Health and Community
Liverpool John Moores University
Henry Cotton Campus
Liverpool, United Kingdom

Jackie Davenport
Faculty of Education, Health and Community
Liverpool John Moores University
Henry Cotton Campus
Liverpool, United Kingdom

Donal Deehan
Faculty of Education, Health and Community
Liverpool John Moores University
Honry Cotton Campus
Liverpool, United Kingdom

Tommy Dunne
Liverpool, United Kingdom

Daz Greenop
Faculty of Education, Health and Community
Liverpool John Moores University
Liverpool, United Kingdom

Julie-Ann Hayes
Faculty of Education, Health and Community
Liverpool John Moores University
Henry Cotton Campus
Liverpool, United Kingdom

James Kidd
Faculty of Education, Health and Community
Liverpool John Moores University
Henry Cotton Campus
Liverpool, United Kingdom

Deborah Knott
Faculty of Education, Health and Community
Liverpool John Moores University
Henry Cotton Campus
Liverpool, United Kingdom

Robert G. MacDonald
Reader in Architecture
Liverpool John Moores University
Liverpool, United Kingdom

Denise Parker
Faculty of Education, Health and Community
Liverpool John Moores University
Henry Cotton Campus
Liverpool, United Kingdom

Rebecca Rylance
Faculty of Education, Health and Community
Liverpool John Moores University
Henry Cotton Campus
Liverpool, United Kingdom

Lorraine Shaw
Faculty of Education, Health and Community
Liverpool John Moores University
Liverpool, United Kingdom

Grahame Smith
Faculty of Education, Health and Community
Liverpool John Moores University
Henry Cotton Campus
Liverpool, United Kingdom

Carol Wilcock
Greater Manchester, United Kingdom

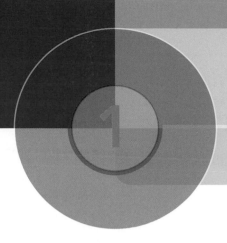

Dementia awareness

SUSAN ASHTON

AIM

- To explore what is meant by dementia awareness

OBJECTIVES

- To identify the main types of dementia and their common features
- To demonstrate an understanding of the different types of treatment options
- To understand the role of the nurse when caring for a person with dementia

OVERVIEW

In the United Kingdom there are approximately 820,000 people with dementia. This number is expected to rise as the population ages and physicians become more skilled in diagnosing dementia. Prior to the 1980s it was not uncommon for older people to be admitted to hospital with a preliminary diagnosis of 'chronic brain failure' or 'senile dementia'. Fortunately, as a result of increased interest in dementia by researchers, clinicians and successive governments, both nationally and internationally, there is a recognition that dementia is a complex disease and not just a consequence of growing older. Dementia has been described as a public health priority by the World Health Organisation (WHO, 2012). The WHO (2012) suggested that further improvements are needed to diagnose, offer treatment options and support people and their carers throughout the dementia journey.

There have been numerous reports from the UK government to identify what the health, care and research priorities should be (HM Government, 2007; Department of Health [DH],

2008, 2009a, 2009b). The National Dementia Strategy was launched to focus on what needs to be done from improved diagnosis to end-of-life care to improve the care and treatment of people with dementia (DH, 2009). It acknowledged a lack of appropriate research, care and treatment and called for a 'transformation' in the quality of care provided to people with dementia and their families or carers (DH, 2009a).

The education of all health and social care staff is also considered a priority to ensure people with a diagnosis of dementia are cared for in an appropriate and supportive way. NHS England has identified minimum standards of education and training with the Department of Health (DH) to familiarise people and raise awareness with recognising and understanding dementia, to interact with those with dementia, and to be able to signpost patients and carers to appropriate support. The learning outcomes for this training must be:

- Better diagnosis, training and care of those with dementia
- Staff will have a greater awareness and confidence to support patients affected by dementia
- Staff will be able to identify the early symptoms of dementia
- Staff will be aware of the needs of patients affected by dementia and their families and carers to enable them to provide safe, dignified and compassionate care
- General practitioners (GPs) will be able to identify and work with patients affected by dementia
- Staff will be able to signpost patients and carers to appropriate support
- Staff will have raised awareness of the increased likelihood of mental health problems in those with long-term conditions

This chapter utilises a scenario-based approach throughout to explore the issues within a practice context.

Rosie is 75 years old. She has always been described as a bit eccentric. She has never followed the crowd. When she was younger, she travelled the world, usually backpacking and taking different jobs as she went along. Her favourite pastimes have included going to Rolling Stones concerts and riding a motorcycle. She married when she was 30 years old and had one child, Sarah. Sarah died of cancer at the age of 31, so Rosie cared for her only grandchild, Jenna, who was 13 years old at the time of Sarah's death. Rosie is now 75 and has always been a bit forgetful and easily distracted. When Jenna points out her recent memory losses Rosie just laughs and says, 'Oh it's just old age'. Jenna is not convinced, but as long as Rosie is happy and managing her own life she is not too worried.

EARLY IDENTIFICATION

Almost all types of dementia are progressive and incurable. The incidence of dementia is similar in men and women (Alzheimer's Society, 2011). However because their life expectancy is greater and age is a risk factor in dementia, more women are likely to have dementia. Early identification of symptoms is important if appropriate treatment and information are to be given to patients. The National Institute for Health and Care Excellence (NICE, 2015c) suggests referring people with mild cognitive impairment for assessment to memory assessment services. This is important for people in high-risk groups such as those people with learning disabilities, those with Parkinson's disease or those who have had a stroke.

Typical symptoms might include (Alzheimer's Society, 2007):

- *Loss of memory.* This is more than just forgetting where you left the car keys. This might include forgetting the way home, inability to recognise and handle money, or being unable to remember names and places.
- *Mood changes.* People with dementia may find it difficult to control their emotions, especially if this area of the brain is affected. They may feel sad, angry, or frightened, which may not necessarily be appropriate to the stimulus (e.g. an irrational fear that someone is going to hurt them).
- *Communication problems.* People with dementia may find it increasingly difficult to talk, read and write and have difficulty with language (e.g. finding the right words for everyday objects such as chair, coat, toilet).

Although some people may be concerned with their symptoms, they might find it difficult to accept a diagnosis of dementia. Alternatively, some people may find it a relief if their recent behaviour has been out of character and they were unable to understand what was happening to them. General practitioners (GPs) are in a good position to identify some of these symptoms if presented by the patient during a consultation. It may be a family member who has recognised something is wrong and has persuaded the person to seek some medical advice. Accurate diagnosis is important to identify the reason for the symptoms and exclude any other cause of the cognitive or memory problems. For example, depression and delirium can sometimes mimic the symptoms of dementia (Weatherhead & Courtney, 2012).

Dementia is a complex disorder and has an unpredictable disease trajectory (Sampson et al., 2008), therefore a patient is often referred to a specialist memory assessment service or memory clinic which often involves a multidisciplinary team of practitioners such as neurologist, psychiatrist, and mental health nurse practitioner.

Nurses working in memory clinics can provide much-needed support and guidance to patients who have recently been diagnosed with dementia and their carers. *Admiral nurses* are specialist dementia nurses who work with families affected by dementia (Harrison-Denning, 2013).

We return to the scenario with Rosie:

Jenna has a very close relationship with her grandmother Rosie. Recently Jenna has become more concerned about Rosie's behaviour. She has always been 'different and unpredictable' but recently Rosie has been calling Jenna up in the middle of the night saying someone is in the house and is trying to attack her. Jenna has always responded and found nothing untoward. In the morning Rosie does not remember the incident and seems just like her old self. Over the next few months Rosie's behaviour continued to be unpredictable and Jenna became more worried. Jenna went to visit Rosie and found the fridge full of broccoli. Rosie just said she liked broccoli and avoided answering any questions on this. Jenna considered taking Rosie to see the GP. One night Rose called Jenna on the telephone screaming that someone was in the house trying to rape her. Jenna quickly went to see Rosie to find no one in the house. However, Rosie appeared confused and disorientated and for a short time did not recognise Jenna. The confusion soon subsided and Rosie settled to sleep. The following day Jenna made an appointment with the GP for Rosie.

ASSESSMENT

Dementia is an umbrella term for a variety of diseases of the brain that are progressive and terminal in nature. Dementia is the term used to describe the symptoms that occur when the brain is affected by certain specific diseases and conditions (Smith & McKenzie, 2011). It is an acquired decline in a range of cognitive abilities (memory, learning, orientation and attention) and intellectual skills (abstraction, judgement, comprehension, language and calculation) accompanied by alterations in personality and behaviour which impair daily functioning social skills and emotional control (Bowie et al., 2004; Phillips, Ajrouch, & Hillcoat-Nalletamby, 2010).

There are potentially 200 different types of dementia. The most common are Alzheimer's disease, vascular dementia, mixed dementia (Alzheimer's and vascular dementia), dementia with Lewy body and fronto-temporal dementia (Pick's disease) (Weatherhead & Courtney, 2012; Smith & McKenzie, 2011). Other dementias include Down's syndrome with dementia and Creutzfeldt-Jakob disease. It is important to exclude acute confusional states and other causes that may mimic the signs of dementia but may be treated successfully (e.g. depression and delirium).

Let us return to Rosie:

The GP was very interested in Jenna's account of Rosie's behaviour. However he said it might be any number of things and the first thing that was needed was a blood test to rule out any underlying cause for the confusion and disorientation. The GP also asked questions about all the incidents that had occurred over the last few months which were 'out of character'. She also asked questions about Rosie's lifestyle and past medical history. She then asked Rosie to complete a short quiz, the Mini-Mental State Examination (MMSE). Rosie refused to take the test, saying she was not 'demented'. However she did agree to the blood test.

A patient presenting with symptoms of dementia will need a comprehensive assessment which should include a detailed account of the person's health and social history. The DH (2011) has issued guidance on the assessment and diagnosis of dementia that emphasises the importance of a broad and comprehensive assessment with the patient and ideally the family carer. When a diagnosis is being made, NICE (2015a, 2015b, 2015c) recommends the dementia pathway:

- Patient is assessed. The MMSE is an example of a validated instrument that is a formal cognitive testing tool as part of a clinical assessment (Folstein, Folstein, & Mchugh, 1975).
- Organise meeting to communicate diagnosis.
- Communicate diagnosis.
- Share information and signpost services.
- Agree and document personalised care plan.
- Organise next meeting.
- Communicate serious illness notification to GP.
- Patient commences support intervention.

The follow-up meeting with the GP was for the results of the blood tests. The tests did not demonstrate anything significant to suggest any underlying condition. This time, Rosie agreed to an MMSE. Rosie continued to exhibit uncharacteristic behaviour. Rosie had always dressed a little differently (never colour coordinated), but she now appeared not to recognise the order in which clothes should be put on. Jenna started calling around every day to see what 'Rosie had done now'. Jenna loved Rosie, but it was becoming hard work and worrying. Rosie just kept saying everything was OK. Rosie still occasionally phoned Jenna in the night saying someone was in the house. One evening, a neighbour of Rosie's called Jenna to say Rosie had been wandering in the street and was extremely agitated and anxious.

CLINICAL FEATURES

Dementia can be associated with a wide variety of changes within the brain. Dementia is an incurable progressive terminal condition (Mitchell et al., 2004) which has an unpredictable disease trajectory (DH, 2009). Dementia often starts gradually and a typical trajectory can last over several years (Phillips, Ajrouch, & Hillcoat-Nalletamby, 2010). The person may initially deny what is happening and make excuses and stories to cover up symptoms. Mild dementia suggests the person can still manage independently, moderate dementia is when some support is needed to perform tasks, and severe dementia is when continual help and support are necessary (Phillips, Ajrouch, & Hillcoat-Nalletamby, 2010).

Life expectancy for people with dementia is dependent on the age at which the disease is first diagnosed and can range from 2 to 10 years (van der Steen et al., 2013). Most people with dementia also have at least one other co-morbidity (National Audit Office, 2007) and often present with complex physical and psychological needs, particularly in the advanced stage of the disease (Sampson et al., 2008).

Alzheimer's disease is the most common cause of dementia and represents approximately 50–60% of cases. Memory disorders are the most common feature. There is a loss of neurons in the temporal lobe and hippocampus, which are the areas of the brain responsible for storing and retrieving new information. The disease also involves the more posterior parts of the brain (parietal lobes), which results in difficulties with language skills (dysphasia) and visuospatial and practical abilities (dyspraxia). If there is also involvement of the frontal lobe of the brain, personality, behaviour, social judgements and insight can be impaired (McKeith & Fairbairn, 2001; Walsh, 2006). The involvement of many different parts of the brain can explain why the symptoms are so varied and complex when considered together. The disease has a gradual onset over several years, with a steady decline in functional abilities.

Mood disorders, anxiety and depression and psychotic symptoms can also present in a number of people (20–40%). This may include hallucinations and delusions, agitation, aggression, sleeping, eating and continence problems, however these generally occur in the later stages of dementia (McKeith & Fairbairn, 2001; Walsh, 2006). It should be remembered that changes in behaviour should always be explored to discover if there is an alternative explanation, such as pain or discomfort due to an underlying or undiagnosed condition.

Vascular dementia can be described as a 'stepwise' progression. The person may experience several episodes which involve a lack of oxygen to the brain, which occur over several months or years and cause 'stepdown' deterioration in ability and cognitive function (McKeith & Fairbairn, 2001; Walsh, 2006). Depending on where the damage is, symptoms may vary amongst individuals; some skills may be lost (e.g. language), but others may remain (e.g. memory).

The brain needs a good supply of oxygen. Vascular is caused when the brain's small blood vessels burst or become blocked, which may be a result of a stroke or several small strokes. A stroke, or cerebrovascular accident (CVA), is when blood does not get to the brain cells. The blood supply is cut off and lack of oxygen causes the death of brain cells. The onset is often sudden and may be followed by further strokes; this is known as multi-infarct dementia (McKeith & Fairbairn, 2001; Walsh, 2006).

Dementia with Lewy bodies is the second most common neurodegenerative disorder after Alzheimer's disease and is defined as a degeneration in the central, peripheral and autonomic nervous system associated with Lewy bodies (Fujishiro et al., 2013). Presenting symptoms include language, concentration and coordination problems which can result in frequent falls. The loss of memory is not as obvious as in other dementias but the person may fluctuate between periods of lucidity and confusion. Auditory and visual hallucinations are common and can be distressing for the patient and the patient's family (McKeith & Fairbairn, 2001; Walsh, 2006).

There are two types of frontal lobe dementia: the frontal type of dementia and the anterior temporal lobe dementia. The frontal type of dementia is characterised by changes in behaviour and is associated with younger age groups (McKeith & Fairbairn, 2001). This can present in a variety of ways such as disinhibition, poor social judgement, and personality changes. Memory and language can be preserved in the early stages. Symptoms associated with the anterior temporal lobe include early loss of language abilities and a loss of understanding of visual and verbal information (McKeith & Fairbairn, 2001).

All these diseases have some similar features: They affect memory, reasoning, communication and mood, and each person's trajectory or journey will be unique (see Table 1.1).

Table 1.1 Features of dementia

Symptom	Example
Deteriorating memory and loss of ability to learn	• Difficulty in remembering recent events • Eventually may be unable to recognise family members and friends • Difficulty in learning new tasks
Loss of orientation skills	• Unable to find own way home • Unable to recognise familiar places
Intellectual decline	• Difficulty in following recent events, understanding situations, reading and writing
Loss of linguistic ability (aphasia)	• Difficulty in finding the right words • Difficulty in forming sentences • Difficulty in understanding what others are saying or in written text • Naming problems
Loss of ability to interpret (agnosia)	• Difficulty in understanding the environment • Decline in ability to recognise objects, sounds and smells
Impaired ability to do practical tasks (apraxia)	• Complex in the person with dementia due to multi-impairment • Deterioration of problem-solving skills
Deterioration in attention	• Difficulty with problem solving and memory • Difficulty with concentration • Easily distracted by noise and other activities

Table 1.1 (*Continued*) Features of dementia

Symptom	Example
Psychological changes	• Anxiety, depression, uncertainty and isolation
	• Everyday activity a challenge
	• Life becomes dangerous and unpredictable
Loss of judgement and changed behaviour	• Occasional loss of inhibition
	• Reaction driven by fear and uncertainty
	• Aggression and threatening behaviour

Taking this into consideration, let us return to Rosie:

Jenna and Rosie returned to the GP, who now referred Rosie to the memory clinic with a provisional diagnosis of Alzheimer's disease. Jenna was very upset but had already considered this. Rosie appeared to take it in her stride and tried to put on a brave face. Rosie decided she needed to make some big decisions and asked Jenna if she would accept power of attorney on her behalf for both financial and welfare needs. Jenna also contacted the Alzheimer's Society for advice and guidance. Jenna and Rosie had a long talk about the future and how they were going to make the best of each day. Jenna told Rosie that she would make sure Rosie remained in her own home for as long as possible and would ensure she lived her life as she always lived, with her Rolling Stones records and lifestyle quirks.

RISK FACTORS

Older age is a risk factor in dementia but is not the cause. Risk factors can depend on the cause. In the UK general population, screening is not carried out for dementia (NICE, 2014a, 2014b, 2014c).

Vascular dementia is associated with stroke and a lack of blood supply to the brain. Reducing the risk of stroke (e.g. regulating blood pressure, stopping smoking, reducing alcohol intake, reducing obesity and encouraging exercise) are important features in a healthy lifestyle. Early identification of people who may be at risk of stroke is an essential feature of modern medicine, however statins and hormone replacement therapy are not considered specific preventive treatments for the primary prevention of dementia (NICE, 2014a, 2014b, 2014c).

Alzheimer's disease has been associated with a genetic predisposition and several genes have now been associated with the development of this type of dementia. However further research is necessary to develop and identify what leads to the development of Alzheimer's disease. People with learning disabilities (e.g. Down's syndrome) are also at risk of developing dementia at a younger age; this also is associated with genetics. Referral to genetic counselling can be made to those thought to have a genetic cause of dementia and their unaffected relatives (NICE, 2014a, 2014b, 2014c).

BEST PRACTICE

Everybody's Business—Integrated Mental Health Services for Older Adults: A Service Development Guide (DH, 2005) called for an integrated approach to health and social care for the planning, implementation and delivery of

- Primary care
- Home care
- Mainstream and specialist day services
- Sheltered and extra-care housing
- Assistive technology and telecare
- Mainstream and specialist residential care
- Intermediate care and rehabilitation
- Care in general hospitals
- Specialist mental health services

Weatherhead and Courtney (2012) suggest that an early diagnosis of dementia can be beneficial for a number of reasons: to enable access to potential treatments, to allow the person to access financial welfare benefits, and to enable access to specialist teams and support services.

Donepezil, galantamine, rivastigmine and memantine are medications currently recommended by NICE (2014b) (see Table 1.2).

The nurse has an important role to play when caring for a patient who has a diagnosis of dementia. The type of dementia diagnosed can often provide some insight into the type of symptoms the patient may experience. A change in environment can often contribute to an exacerbation of symptoms, for example the patient may become agitated or disorientated.

Each person with dementia is unique, and although some symptoms are common to all, no two people experience dementia in the same way. People with dementia need to feel valued and respected.

Good nursing practice in dementia care includes the following:

- Always address the client in a manner they prefer and recognise.
- Involve family and friends in assessment and encourage an open visiting approach as much as possible. Family and friends can provide essential information and interpretation of the patient's behaviour, likes and dislikes.
- Perform complete risk assessment to identify any potential immediate risks to the patient's safety. This should include the risk to personal and environmental safety.
- Involve medical staff in assessment and be prepared to be an advocate for the patient.
- Allow the patient to settle into the environment. Do not overload the patient with information.

Table 1.2 NICE recommendations

Donepezil	Acetylcholinesterase (AChE) inhibitors
Galantamine	recommended as options for managing
Rivastigmine	mild-to-moderate Alzheimer's disease
Memantine	Recommended as an option for managing Alzheimer's disease for people with moderate disease who cannot take AChE inhibitors or have severe Alzheimer's disease

Treatment should be continued only when it is considered to be having a worthwhile effect on cognitive, global, functional or behavioural symptoms.

Patient's status should be reviewed regularly using cognitive, global, functional and behavioural assessment.

Treatment should be reviewed by an appropriate specialist team unless there are locally agreed-upon protocols for shared care. It is also important to seek carer's views of the patient's condition.

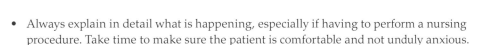

- Always explain in detail what is happening, especially if having to perform a nursing procedure. Take time to make sure the patient is comfortable and not unduly anxious.
- Respect any cultural values and differences. Customs and rules may need to be explained so misunderstandings are minimal.
- Ensure any special needs are considered (e.g. sensory or physical disability).
- Make sure there is sufficient light to ensure good visibility.
- Try to maintain a quiet atmosphere. A noisy environment can be challenging to the person with dementia. This can create fear and anxiety, which may lead to increased agitation and aggression.
- Include familiar objects (e.g. family photographs) in the immediate environment. These can be reassuring to the patient.
- Make sure there are clear orientation signs if the environment is unfamiliar. Words as well as signs can be helpful for the patient with dementia. Colour coordinated doors are also useful (e.g. toilet doors are painted all the same colour).
- Liaise with medical staff to regularly review medication and exclude underlying causes of any changes in behaviour or condition. A sudden increase in symptoms is unlikely to be caused by the dementia.
- Develop an understanding of the person's life history. This is essential to person centred care. Try to get to know your patient's background and history. This can help when trying to understand behaviour or what the person may need.
- Establish a usual routine and habitual behaviour. Try to keep to the patient's usual routine and daily activities. Maintain and promote functional ability as much as possible.
- Keep family and friends informed concerning medical/nursing care. This can avoid misunderstandings and reduce any anxieties they may have. Family members may have been caring for the person for several years and will find it difficult to relinquish their role to a health professional, so it is important to respect their knowledge and understanding of the person with dementia.
- If the patient becomes agitated, your approach should be to reduce the agitation. Try to find out what might have triggered the behavioural change. Be calm and talk quietly to the patient and do not challenge or argue with the patient. It may be helpful to redirect attention (e.g. offer a cup of tea).
- In discussions with the patient, colleagues and family, establish an appropriate level of observation. It may not be suitable to isolate the patient in a side room, as this may cause the patient to become further disorientated and anxious. However a side room may provide quiet space in a busy ward environment.
- Always record and report the patient's behaviour each shift or visit. This is important to observe any triggers which may cause the patient to be anxious or agitated so these can be avoided or anticipated in the future. For example, if taking the patient's blood pressure triggers an aggressive response this can be anticipated so that more care and time can be utilised to facilitate this procedure.

We now return to Rosie:

Rosie's diagnosis was confirmed as Alzheimer's disease. Treatment options were discussed at the memory clinic and information given regarding how Rosie and Jenna could prepare for the future. Jenna had found a support group and received some information from Age UK and the Alzheimer's Society. At present Rosie was doing fine; she was still able to live independently, but Jenna was visiting more often and sometimes staying overnight. Rosie's next door neighbour was willing to help and keep an eye on her, especially during the early evening. Jenna was now looking into assistive technologies in anticipation of any future deterioration in Rosie's mental state. Rosie and Jenna were taking each day as it came and had been making the most of life. They had decided to book a short holiday to Spain.

CAPACITY

The Mental Capacity Act (MCA, 2005) came into force in 2007. The assumption should always be that the person has capacity to make their own decisions unless they have been assessed as not having capacity.

If an assessment of incapacity is made the person will not be able to do the following (MCA, 2005):

- Understand the information relevant to the decision
- Retain information for long enough periods to make a decision on it
- Use the information in their decision-making
- Communicate their decision

People with dementia may be assumed to lack capacity but this should not be the case. The nurse should always assume initially that the person has capacity and that the person is capable of giving consent. If a person has been assessed as lacking capacity, it may be 'at this time' as people with dementia can sometimes have fluctuating capacity. If decisions are made for the person who lacks capacity, these must be in the person's best interest and be the least restrictive.

As the disease progresses, a family caregiver or representative may apply for lasting power of attorney (LPA). Sometimes this has already been organised when the person with dementia was initially diagnosed and appointed the person they most wanted to make decisions on their behalf. An LPA is a legal document that allows the designated person to act as an 'attorney' to make decisions in relation to financial affairs or personal welfare on behalf of a person who may lack the mental capacity to do so himself. An LPA must be registered with the Office of the Public Guardian in order to be legal (Barber, Brown, & Martin, 2012; HM Government, 2012).

CHAPTER SUMMARY

Dementia is a complex disease. Each person who has dementia will experience it in a unique way. An individualised assessment is essential to ensure an accurate diagnosis and treatment plan.

Dementia can take several years to develop, so it is important to have an understanding of the common features of the disease and not dismiss them as being a part of old age.

Whatever the stage of the disease, the nurse needs an appreciation of how dementia can influence a patient's response to being cared for.

The caring environment can be stressful for a person with dementia so the nurse needs to undertake a detailed individualised assessment involving the patient and the family caregivers.

REFLECTION ON LEARNING

1. What is dementia?
2. Why is it important to diagnose dementia early in the disease?
3. What are three typical features of dementia?
4. What is a memory clinic?
5. What is the MMSE?
6. What are the main types of dementia?
7. What are the risk factors associated with dementia?
8. When might treatment be discontinued in dementia?
9. What must you consider when caring for a person with dementia?
10. What is a lasting power of attorney?

REFERENCES

Alzheimer's Society. 2007. *The Rising Cost of Dementia in the UK*. London: London School of Economics and the Institute of Psychiatry.

Alzheimer's Society. 2011. *What Is Dementia?* London: London School of Economics and the Institute of Psychiatry.

Barber, P., Brown, R., & Martin, D. 2012. *Mental Health Law in England and Wales. A Guide for Mental Health Professionals*, 2nd edition. London: Sage.

Department of Health. 2005. *Everybody's Business—Integrated Mental Health Services for Older Adults with Mental Health Problems: A Service Development Guide*. London: Department of Health.

Department of Health. 2008. *Transforming the Quality of Dementia Care: Consultation on a National Dementia Strategy*. London: Department of Health.

Department of Health. 2009a. *Living Well with Dementia: A National Dementia Strategy*. London: DH.

Department of Health. 2009b. *Living Well with Dementia: A National Dementia Strategy—Implementation Plan*. London: Department of Health.

Department of Health. 2011. *Service Specification for Dementia: Memory Service for Early Diagnosis and Intervention*. London: Department of Health.

Folstein, M.F., Folstein, S.E., & Mchugh, P.R. 1975. 'Mini mental state': A practical method for grading the cognitive state of the patient for the clinician. *Journal of Psychiatric Research* 12(3): 189–198.

Fujishiro, H., Isekl, E., Nakamura, S., Kasanuki, K., Chiba, Y., Ota, K., Murayama, N., & Sato, K. 2013. Dementia with Lewy bodies: Early diagnostic challenges. *Psychogeriatrics*, 13: 128–138.

Gundy, E. 2006. Ageing and vulnerable elderly people: European perspective. *Ageing & Society*, 26: 105–134.

Harrison-Denning, K. 2013. Dementia: Diagnosis and early interventions. *British Journal of Nursing*, 9(3): 131–137.

HM Government. 2007. *Putting People First: A Shared Vision and Commitment to the Transformation of Adult Social Care*. London: HM Government.

HM Government. 2012. Make, Register or End a Lasting Power of Attorney. https://www.gov.uk/power-of-attorney.

McKeith, I., & Fairbairn, A. 2001. Biomedical and clinical perspectives. In *A Handbook of Dementia Care*, edited by Cantley, C., 7–27. Buckingham, UK: Open University Press.

Mitchell, S.L., Morris, J.N., Park, P.S., & Fries, B.E. 2004. Terminal care for persons with advanced dementia in the nursing home and home care settings. *Journal of Palliative Medicine*, 7(6): 808–816.

National Audit Office. 2007. *Improving Services and Support for People with Dementia*. London: NAO.

National Institute for Health and Care Excellence. 2015a. Dementia Diagnosis and Assessment. http://pathways.nice.org.uk/pathways/dementia#path=view%3A/pathways/dementia/dementia-diagnosis-and-assessment.xml&content=view-index.

National Institute for Health and Care Excellence. 2015b. Dementia Interventions. http://pathways.nice.org.uk/pathways/dementia#path=view%3A/pathways/dementia/dementia-interventions.xml&content=view-index.

National Institute for Health and Care Excellence. 2015c. Dementia Overview. http://pathways.nice.org.uk/pathways/dementia.

Phillips, J., Ajrouch, K., & Hillcoat-Nalletamby, S. 2010. *Key Concepts in Social Gerontology*. London: Sage.

Sampson, E.L., Thune-Boyle, I., Kukkastenvehmas, R., Jones, L., Tookman, A., King, M., & Blanchard, M.R. 2008. Palliative care in advanced dementia: A mixed methods approach for the development of a complex intervention. *BMC Palliative Care*, 7(8). doi:10.1186/1472-684X-7-8.

Smith, K.T., & McKenzie, L. 2011. Dementia: Complex case work. In *Mental Health and Later Life. Delivering a Holistic Model for Practice*, edited by Keady, J., & Watts, S., 137–152. Abingdon, UK: Routledge.

Van der Steen, J.T., Radbruch, L., Hertogh, C.M.P.M., de Boar, M.E., Hughes, J.C., Larkin, P., Volicer, L., on behalf of the European Association for Palliative Care. 2013. White paper defining optimal palliative care in older people with dementia: A Delphi Study and recommendations from the EACP. *Palliative Medicine*, 28(3) 197–209.

Walsh, D. 2006. *Dementia Care Training Manual for Staff Working in Nursing and Residential Settings*. London: Kingsley.

Weatherhead, I., & Courtney, C. 2012. Assessing the signs of dementia. *Practice Nursing*, 23(3): 114–119.

World Health Organisation. 2012. *Dementia. A Public Health Priority*. Geneva: WHO.

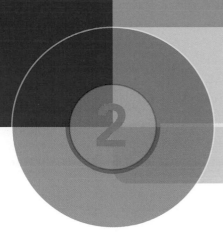

Social policy and dementia

LORRAINE SHAW AND DENISE PARKER

AIM

- To reflect on social policy within a dementia context

OBJECTIVES

- To consider the impact of demographic change and how societies are responding
- To examine in depth the notion of 'dementia-friendly' communities
- To think about living well with dementia as a health promotion strategy
- To identify the successes and the challenges of the commissioning process

OVERVIEW

As people are living longer, it is predicted that the prevalence of people with dementia will increase (Woods et al., 2013). Dementia is a long-term condition that adversely impacts a person's cognitive abilities, emotional and behavioural control, and social functioning above and beyond what might be expected from normal aging (Woods et al., 2013). Currently it is estimated there are 35.6 million people worldwide with dementia; this number is expected to double by 2030 and potentially more than triple by 2050 (WHO, 2012; Woods et al., 2013). Globally it is recognised that there is still much to be done:

> Dementia is overwhelming not only for the people who have it, but also for their caregivers and families. It is one of the major causes of disability and dependency among older people worldwide. There is lack of awareness and understanding of dementia, at some level, in most countries, resulting in stigmatization, barriers to diagnosis and care, and impacting

caregivers, families and societies physically, psychologically and economically. Dementia can no longer be neglected but should be considered a part of the public health agenda in all countries. (WHO, 2012: 2)

With this growing recognition there is an acceptance that to meet this increasing demand societies must look for innovative solutions (Woods et al., 2013). A starting place is to ensure that dementia stops being a 'hidden illness' and that people with dementia and their carers at the point of diagnosis have timely access to sufficient information and advice and a clear and supportive pathway of care from diagnosis to end-of-life care (Prince, Bryce, & Ferri, 2011; Woods et al., 2013; Alzheimer's Society, 2013, 2014). Receiving a timely diagnosis of dementia can be a challenge:

Ensuring a timely, quality diagnosis of dementia must remain a priority in the UK. Many people are getting the diagnosis they need too late or not at all. In the UK, diagnosis rates range from less than 40% to over 75%. (Alzheimer's Society, 2014: 6)

The importance of receiving an early diagnosis is that a person and his or her carers can in theory access the services they require (Alzheimer's Society, 2014). As with the drive to improve access to an early diagnosis, there is a similar ambition to increase the choice of services available for people living with dementia and to improve the quality-of-care outcomes for both existing and future services (Department of Health [DH], 2009, 2011; Alzheimer's Society, 2014). To consider in more depth the issues that arise, this chapter explores and develops the following scenario:

Mr Walker is 72 years old and has been living well with dementia for approximately 5 years. His wife of 50 years is his primary carer, and his large extended family are very supportive. Mr Walker was diagnosed by his general practitioner (GP) with mixed dementia but receives no organised support. Until recently, Mr Walker was able to walk unaided to his local betting shop and attended family functions. Recently and quite suddenly, Mr Walker's condition started to deteriorate. His memory has declined, he can no longer go out unaided, he has some problems with continence, and his sleep is severely disrupted—he often wanders around the house at night. In addition, his wife was recently diagnosed with terminal cancer. Understandably, she is not coping. The family stepped in to provide full-time care to their parents. After 2 weeks, the family is exhausted and desperate; they consider taking Mr Walker to the accident and emergency (A&E) department.

A SOCIETAL RESPONSE

Globally, the population is aging rapidly; it is predicted that by 2050 people aged over 60 will account for 22% of the world's population, compared to current figures of 8%. This will significantly increase the number of individuals living with dementia (WHO, 2012). It was also estimated in 2011 that globally there were 35.6 million people with dementia; it is projected that there will be an increase to 65.7 million in 2030 and 115.4 million in 2050 (Woods et al., 2013; WHO, 2012). Within a UK context:

There are 835,000 people living with dementia in the UK in 2014, and by 2015 that figure will be 850,000. It is the most feared health condition for people over the age of 55, but touches people of all ages. Over 21 million people know close friends or family affected by the condition. Dementia costs the UK economy over £26 billion per year—higher than cancer, heart disease or stroke. (Alzheimer's Society, 2014: Foreword)

Estimates for dementia are based on the premise that the risk of dementia increases with age. As it is projected that more and more societies will have aging populations, there is then an expectation that not only will dementia rates increase but rates of people with the later stages of dementia will increase as well (Woods et al., 2013; WHO, 2012). Measuring and comparing prevalence rates across societies is a challenge, as reporting mechanisms vary from country to country. Taking Europe as a whole, WHO (2012) indicated that the prevalence of dementia was 0.9% for people aged 60–64, 1.3% for those aged 65–69, 3.3% for those aged 70–74, 5.8% for individuals aged 75–79, 12.3% for those aged 80–84, and 24.6% for people aged 85 and above. Within the UK the prevalence rates are similar, although the Alzheimer's Society (2014) suggested that due to improvements in treating underlying vascular problems some age-related prevalence rates have decreased. For certain groups of people who are now living longer, including people with Down's syndrome, learning disabilities, and Parkinson's disease and those who have had a stroke, the prevalence of dementia is increasing (Woods et al., 2013).

It is generally recognised that for the older adult dementia is one of the main causes of disability. The findings from the United Nations summit (2011) highlight that neurological disorders such as dementia are a major cause of morbidity and that they have a significant social and economic impact (Woods et al., 2013; United Nations, 2011). The declaration emanating from the summit urged governments to take responsibility by engaging with all their citizens in the process of providing health and social care interventions in an effective and equitable way that support people living with dementia (Woods et al., 2013; United Nations, 2011).

Providing services that reach all sections of society is a challenge. Within the UK there is an expectation that incidents of dementia will rise more sharply within black and minority ethnic communities (Woods et al., 2013; DH, 2009). This may in part be due to people from black and minority ethnic communities historically having a low presentation to services although in some cases they may have higher rates of dementia. As awareness increases and potentially presentation rates increase, this could in turn lead to a sharp rise of identified cases (Mukadam, Cooper, & Livingston, 2011). Increasing awareness of dementia within black and minority ethnic communities is a good starting place to ensure that services are then fit for purpose, but there has to be a concerted effort to improve access to services, increase the quality of support available, and to fund research that robustly identifies the specific needs and preferences of people living with dementia (Woods et al., 2013; Moriarty, Sharif, & Robinson, 2011).

Dementia has a financial cost to society:

The total estimated worldwide costs of dementia were US$604 billion in 2010. In high-income countries, informal care (45%) and formal social care (40%) account for the majority of costs, while the proportionate contribution of direct medical costs (15%) is much lower. (WHO, 2012: 2)

Within Europe, the cost of dementia is estimated to be 130 billion euros a year, which includes both direct and indirect costs (European Commission and Economic Policy Committee, 2009; Wimo, Winbladand, & Jonsson, 2010; Woods et al., 2013). As dementia is age related, these costs are expected to increase. Within a UK context, the population in 2012 was approximately

62.3 million, and by 2050 the population is estimated to be 78.7 million; the proportion of people aged 65 and over is also expected to increase significantly. The cost of dementia is predicted to increase from over £20 billion a year to over £50 billion a year (Woods et al., 2013; Office for National Statistics, 2012; Comas-Herrera et al., 2007).

Within the United Kingdom, the majority of people with dementia live in their own homes. In addition, there are an estimated 670,000 primary carers who deliver informal care, which is estimated to save the UK economy £11 billion per year (Alzheimer's Society, 2013, 2014). In terms of residential or hospital care, dementia is a 'strong pre-determinant' for admission; similarly, when admitted to a hospital, people with dementia occupy up to a quarter of the beds at any one time (Woods et al., 2013; Forma et al., 2011; Alzheimer's Society 2009).

To meet these social challenges, the United Kingdom has developed a number of dementia strategies, which include the following: *Living Well with Dementia: A National Dementia Strategy for England* (DH, 2009); *Improving Dementia Services in Northern Ireland: A Regional Strategy* (Department of Health, Social Services and Public Safety [DHSSPS], 2011); *National Dementia Vision for Wales* (Welsh Assembly Government, 2011); and *Scotland's National Dementia Strategy: 2013–2016* (Scottish Government, 2013). All of these strategies to a greater or lesser degree aim to promote dementia awareness within society as a whole, increase early diagnosis and treatment rates, and improve the provision of good-quality care from diagnosis to the end of life (Woods et al., 2013). In addition, there is a need to improve investment in dementia research, with investment being relatively low compared to other long-term conditions (Luengo-Fernandez, Leal, & Gray, 2010; Woods et al., 2013). The prime minister's challenge initiatives are an example of building these strategies on the inclusion of a focus on the need for investment in research funding (DH, 2012, 2015). The dementia challenge initiative from 2012 was updated in early 2015; it set out a programme of work with an ambition for England to be 'the best country in the world for dementia care and support, and the best place in the world to undertake research into dementia' (DH, 2015: 2). Let us return to the chapter scenario:

After being referred to a social worker and community psychiatric nurse, the family requested a night-time sitting service and made enquiries about keeping their parents together. However, neither of these could be financially supported; the social worker was concerned about Mr Walker's increasing care needs. Following a review meeting, Mr Walker was admitted for respite and assessment to a residential care home that provides dementia care. Several weeks later, Mr Walker remains in care; however, his condition has markedly deteriorated. He has lost weight, has become very agitated, and is described by care staff as aggressive at times, although the family have seen no evidence of this. Mr Walker is distressed when his family visits, and he asks to go home.

DEMENTIA-FRIENDLY COMMUNITIES

Projects are now underway across the UK with the ambition of making our communities easier places for people affected by dementia to access services, socialise and live well. (Alzheimer's Society, 2014: Executive Summary)

Dementia-friendly communities are not only about good design but also relate to people with dementia feeling part of the wider community (Alzheimer's Society, 2014). Environments of good design that are calming, safe and understandable can have a positive impact on the quality of life of a person with dementia by reducing agitation and confusion (Woods et al., 2013; Zeisel et al., 2003; Lawton, 2001). On this basis, the principles of dementia-friendly environments are widely recognised as essential when designing nursing home, hospital, and residential care facilities (Woods et al., 2013; Bicket et al., 2010; Marshall 2012; Chaudhury & Cooke, 2014). It is difficult to specifically pin down what exactly constitutes a dementia-friendly environment. Especially where there are many interacting factors involved, design principles help; however, it is also important to understand on a person-centred level how a person interacts with the environment both as an individual and as a member of a community (Woods et al., 2013; Henwood & Downs, 2014). At a general level, recent innovations that have been used to improve the environment for people with dementia include intelligent lighting systems, memory-enabling apps, exercise and nutrition programmes, and the use of colour and imagery in care environments (Woods et al., 2013).

Physical environments are a key part of dementia-friendly communities, as is access to local facilities, support networks, social networks, and local groups (Henwood & Downs, 2014). One way of achieving this is to raise awareness amongst local communities about the challenges of living with dementia and also encourage those members of the community to take action through such initiatives as the 'Dementia Friends' scheme (Woods et al., 2013; DH, 2009). At a policy level, 'national plans' have driven the move towards dementia-friendly communities specifically from a social inclusion perspective (Henwood & Downs, 2014). This move is based on the view that traditional models of care need to change and be more focused on citizenship and social inclusion (Woods et al., 2013). The impact on contemporary health and social care delivery is that there is more acceptance that care should be individualised, personalised, accessible, and flexible with a focus on more choice (Woods et al., 2013).

To drive this change within health-care settings, a system of improvement targets and key priorities is used, such as ensuring every person over the age of 75 admitted to a hospital has his or her 'memory checked' and early diagnosis is prioritised; that staff have the right skills and the right support to effectively care for people with dementia; and that the environment is dementia friendly (DH, 2009, 2011; Royal College of Nursing, 2013; National Institute for Health and Care Excellence [NICE], 2007). We now return to the scenario:

After spending time with his family, Mr Walker appears more relaxed and less confused; he agrees to stay. His family is concerned about his level of confusion, and after searching the web they return to the home and ask the following questions (Chaudhury & Cooke, 2014):

- Could the environment be more homelike?
- Can they bring in some of Mr Walker's personal belongings?
- Are the staff Dementia Friends?

LIVING WELL

Globally, dementia is a public health priority; certainly, within the United Kingdom there is a drive to increase dementia awareness throughout society with a focus on supporting people to live well with dementia. There is more work to be done, including continuing the work on increasing public awareness, tackling fear and stigma, promoting early diagnosis, and reducing social isolation (WHO, 2012; DH, 2009; DHSSPS, 2011; Welsh Assembly Government, 2011; Scottish Government, 2013; National Collaborating Centre for Mental Health [NCCMH], 2007/2011; Alzheimer's Society, 2013).

Living well with dementia relates not only to promotion but also to prevention, which includes a societal focus on the development, initiation, and monitoring of prevention strategies (WHO, 2012; Ballenger, 2014). At this junction stage, it is important to note that a 'cause' for dementia (Alzheimer's) has not been identified, and that the research evidence on prevention is still in an early stage (WHO, 2012). Even so, there is sufficient evidence available to inform the types of prevention strategies that could reduce risk; these strategies can also be used as strategies for living well. These strategies include supporting people to (WHO, 2012):

- Stop smoking
- Eat a balanced diet
- Be health screened
- Reduce weight where required
- Engage in activities that maintain a healthy heart
- Keep physically and mentally active

The emphasis on health promotion and prevention has underpinned the societal move from just controlling the symptoms of dementia to focusing more on improving the quality of life and well-being for people living with dementia (DH, 2009; DHSSPS, 2011; Welsh Assembly Government, 2011; Scottish Government, 2013). This approach will only work effectively where there is a concerted effort to really understand the individual's needs and challenges, both as a person with dementia and as a person who is an informal carer (Kitwood, 1997; Woods, 2004). Indeed, policy within the United Kingdom is committed to this person-centred approach, although there is more work to be done to ensure that health and social care delivery offers support and interventions that improve the quality of life of people living with dementia in all situations (DH, 2009; DHSSPS, 2011; Welsh Assembly Government, 2011; Scottish Government, 2013; Alzheimer's Society, 2014).

Person-centred care is a 'working with' arrangement, and on this basis there is a need to strengthen the rights of people living with dementia so they feel empowered as active partners within the care delivery process (Mast, 2014). Not enough consideration is given to the rights of people living with dementia; some of this stems from a lack of knowledge about dementia and its relationship to a person's rights in society (European Commission, 2009; Alzheimer's Society, 2014; DH, 2005). Within the UK, the emphasis on promoting dementia awareness as both health and social care training issues will in part address this concern (DH, 2014, 2015). In addition, there is a need to strengthen these initiatives. The introduction of changes to the law regarding human rights and capacity and changes to the way health and social care are delivered with more of a focus on maximising independence is seen as a step in the right direction (Human Rights Act, 1998; DH, 2005; Care Act, 2014; Alzheimer's Society, 2014). Adhering to the principles of person-centred care will not only empower people living with dementia but also will help to maximise independence by valuing the contribution of people living with dementia, listening to and respecting their unique experiences, and prioritising their right to live well with dementia (Kitwood, 1997; Woods et al., 2013; Mast, 2014; DH, 2009; DHSSPS, 2011; Welsh Assembly Government, 2011; Scottish Government, 2013; Alzheimer's Society, 2014).

The majority of people with dementia 'age in place'—most live at home until the end of life or circumstances change and they need to be admitted to residential care. Sometimes living at home is a choice, although sometimes because of risk this choice is overridden (Woods et al.,

2013; Charlesworth, 2014; DH, 2009). To help people with dementia stay at home as long as possible, personalised home care can be provided that assists a person with dementia to meet his or her daily needs. This includes the preparation and eating of meals, personal hygiene, and going to the toilet (Charlesworth, 2014; Alzheimer's Society, 2014). Assisted technologies can also be provided that enable a person with dementia to do a daily task that, due to the person's condition, the person has been unable to do, such as remembering to take medication or to eat or calling for help if in difficulty (Gibson et al., 2014). The advent of personal care budgets are intended to support these developments; unfortunately. the majority of people with dementia and their carers are not accessing these budgets (Alzheimer's Society, 2014).

If a person with dementia cannot live at home and is admitted to a hospital or residential care, there still is the societal imperative to ensure that the person is supported to live well with maximised independence (DH, 2009; DHSSPS, 2011; Welsh Assembly Government, 2011; Scottish Government, 2013; Alzheimer's Society, 2014). Environments can be changed physically to be more dementia friendly; it is just as important that the culture within hospitals and residential care is also dementia friendly and that care staff have the appropriate training and the motivation to be dementia friendly (Davis et al., 2009; Calkins, 2009; DH, 2014, 2015). The chapter scenario addresses these points:

The care manager recognised that there was more work to be done: The physical environment could be made more homelike, and the family could bring in some of Mr Walker's personal belongings. Some, but not all, of the staff had undergone dementia awareness training, and this needed to be addressed. The family felt reassured that they were being listened to, however they were keen that action was taken. Over a 3-month period of time, Mr Walker's behaviour continued to be cyclic. There was no evidence of agitation when his family visited, although staff still reported he would become very agitated and sometimes aggressive. The family noted during this time that the agreed-upon actions had not taken place and the care manager had left.

COMMISSIONING AND FUNDING

The NHS England and NHS Improving Quality (2014) report, *Dementia Diagnosis and Care in England—Learning from Clinical Commissioning Groups*, highlights the commissioning strategies that are currently working well, including the following:

- The formation of strong working relationships across health and social care that are supported by joint dementia strategies
- The delivery of dementia training programmes across health and social care
- The creation of postdiagnostic support groups, including dementia cafes
- Redesigning of memory services, which includes the offer of home-based assessments
- Better care coordination across services
- A reduction in the use of antipsychotics

The challenges are also highlighted in this report; they include

- Low levels of self-referral for a memory assessment
- GPs not always referring for memory assessment
- Local assessment and referral pathways not always clearly articulated

- Pressure and responsibilities preventing some primary care services being able to manage following up noncomplex cases transferred back to primary care
- Not always sure how to best manage patients with Korsakoff's syndrome
- A lack in some areas of local support for people with early onset dementia
- Within care homes not all staff receive dementia training, and where they do it does not always cover topics such as advance care planning and end-of-life care

Forecasting what services will and should look like is crucial to successful commissioning. The problem is that unknown factors such as new advances in medicine can completely reshape a forecast by dramatically reducing or increasing costs (Woods et al., 2013; Ham, Dixon, & Brooke, 2012). In the meantime, the commissioning process has to deal with the status quo that the prevalence of people with dementia will continue to increase and services need to be resourced and prepared accordingly (WHO, 2012; Alzheimer's Society, 2014). Funding also needs to extend to spending more money in the area of research; funding in this area is still significantly below the money spent on other conditions. For example, 12 times more money is spent on cancer research than on dementia (DH, 2015; Alzheimer's Society, 2014). Returning to the scenario:

Three months later, the care home stated they were unable to meet Mr Walker's care needs and served a notice of eviction. The community psychiatric nurse and social worker applied for Continuing Healthcare Funding (fully funded NHS care) as it was felt Mr Walker's dementia had rapidly deteriorated and he needed elderly mentally ill care. The application for funding was rejected—the local authority disagreed with the assessment of care needs. One month after eviction was served, the family was anxious about what would happen to Mr Walker; they feared they may have to resort to attending A&E, as no alternative care home had been found. On the final day of notice, solicitors agreed eviction was not lawful, and the care home allowed Mr Walker to remain for a few more days. Financial support was put in place to provide extra care until a suitable care home could be found. A week later, Mr Walker was transferred to another care home which had a dementia-friendly strategy in place. Subsequently, Mr Walker started to gain weight and there were no reports of aggressive and agitated behaviour, much to his family's relief.

CHAPTER SUMMARY

The global population is aging rapidly; as a result, the number of people with dementia will significantly increase. These demographic changes and increases are being mirrored within a UK context.

Societies and communities have to be more dementia friendly so people living with dementia feel part of the wider community. Dementia friendly at a micro level relates to good design principles: Residential care environments should be calming, safe, and understandable.

Dementia is a public health priority; on this basis, there is a drive to increase dementia awareness with a focus on supporting people to live well with dementia. There is also a move towards considering dementia within a health prevention context.

The majority of people with dementia live at home. To help people with dementia stay at home as long as safely possible and with a good quality of life, personalised care can be provided; however, the funding for this type of care is not always accessed.

There is much work still to be done. In the area of commissioning dementia care, there are a number of strategies that are working well, although there are still a number of challenges that need to be overcome.

REFLECTION ON LEARNING

1. Globally, how many people are estimated to have dementia, and what will this figure look like in 2050?
2. Dementia is one of the main causes of what in the older adult?
3. To ensure that dementia services are fit for purpose in black and minority ethnic communities, for what does there have to be a concerted effort?
4. Where do the majority of people with dementia live in the United Kingdom?
5. How many primary carers are there in the United Kingdom, and how much is it estimated they save the UK economy?
6. Name the dementia strategies for each UK country.
7. For what are the principles of dementia-friendly environments widely recognised as essential?
8. What are the key components of dementia-friendly communities?
9. In terms of health promotion and prevention, what should health and social practitioners support people to do?
10. Commissioning strategies that are currently working well include which strategies?

REFERENCES

Alzheimer's Society. 2009. *Counting the Cost: Caring for People with Dementia on Hospital Wards*. London: Alzheimer's Society.

Alzheimer's Society. 2013. *Dementia 2013: The Hidden Voice of Loneliness*. London: Alzheimer's Society.

Alzheimer's Society 2014. *Dementia 2014: Opportunity for Change*. London: Alzheimer's Society.

Ballenger, J.F. 2014. Dementia as a public health issue: Research or services? In *Excellence in Dementia Care*, 2nd edition, edited by Downs, M., & Bowers, B., 66–77. Maidenhead, UK: Open University Press.

Bicket, M.C., Quincy, M.S., McNabney, M., Onyike, C.U., Mayer, L.S., Brandt, J., Rabins, P., Lykestos, C., & Rosenblatt, A. 2010. The physical environment influences neuropsychiatric symptoms and other outcomes in assisted living residents. *International Journal of Geriatric Psychiatry*, 25(10): 1044–1054.

Calkins, M.P. 2009. Evidence-based long term care design. *NeuroRehabilitation*, 25: 145–154.

Care Act 2014: Elizabeth II. 2014. Chapter 23. London: Stationery Office.

Chaudhury, H., & Cooke, H. 2014. Design matters in dementia care: The role of the physical environment in dementia care settings. In *Excellence in Dementia Care*, 2nd edition, edited by Downs, M., & Bowers, B., 144–158. Maidenhead, UK: Open University Press.

Charlesworth, G. 2014. Living at home. In *Excellence in Dementia Care*, 2nd edition, edited by Downs, M., & Bowers, B., 303–314. Maidenhead, UK: Open University Press.

Comas-Herrera, A., Wittenberg, R., Pickard, L., & Knapp, M. 2007. Cognitive impairment in older people: Its implications for future demand for services and costs. *International Journal of Geriatric Psychiatry*, 22(10): 1037–1045.

Davis, S., Byers, S., Nay, R., & Koch, S. 2009. Guiding design of dementia friendly environments in residential care settings: Considering the living experiences. *Dementia*, 8(2): 185–203.

Department of Health. 2005. *Mental Capacity Act*. London: HMSO.

Department of Health. 2009. *Living Well with Dementia: A National Dementia Strategy*. London: Department of Health.

Department of Health. 2010. *Nothing Ventured, Nothing Gained: Risk Guidance for People with Dementia*. London: Department of Health.

Department of Health. 2011. *NHS Operating Framework 2012–13*. London: Department of Health.

Department of Health. 2012. *Prime Minister's Challenge on Dementia: Delivering Major Improvements in Dementia Care and Research by 2015*. London: Department of Health.

Department of Health. 2014. *Delivering High Quality, Effective, Compassionate Care: Developing the Right People with the Right Skills and the Right Values—A Mandate from the Government to Health Education England: April 2014 to March 2015*. London: Department of Health.

Department of Health. 2015. *Prime Minister's Challenge on Dementia 2020*. London: Department of Health.

Department of Health, Social Services and Public Safety. 2011. *Improving Dementia Services in Northern Ireland: A Regional Strategy*. Belfast, Northern Ireland: DHSSPS.

European Commission. 2009. *Communication from the Commission to the European Parliament and the Council: On a European Initiative on Alzheimer's Disease and Other Dementias*. Brussels, Belgium: European Commission.

European Commission and Economic Policy Committee. 2009. *2009 Ageing Report: Economic and Budgetary Projections for the EU-27 Member States (2008–2060)*. Luxembourg: Publications Office of the European Union.

Forma, L., Rissanen, P., Aaltonen, M., Raitanen, J., & Jylhä, M. 2011. Dementia as a determinant of social and health service use in the last two years of life 1996–2003. *BMC Geriatrics*, 11(14). doi:10.1186/1471-2318-11-14.

Gibson, G., Newton, L., Pritchard, G., Finch, T., Brittain, K., & Robinson, L. 2014. The provision of assistive technology products and services for people with dementia in the United Kingdom. *Dementia*, 0(0): 1–21. doi:10.1177/1471301214532643.

Ham, C., Dixon, A., & Brooke, B. 2012. *Transforming the Delivery of Health and Social Care*. London: Kings Fund.

Henwood, C., & Downs, M. 2014. Dementia-friendly communities. In *Excellence in Dementia Care*, 2nd edition, edited by Downs, M., & Bowers, B., 20–35. Maidenhead, England: Open University Press.

Human Rights Act 1998: Elizabeth ll. 1988. Chapter 42. London: Stationery Office.

Kitwood, T. 1997. *Dementia Reconsidered*. London: Open University Press.

Lawton, M.P. 2001. The physical environment of the person with Alzheimer's disease. *Aging & Mental Health*, 5(supplement 1): 56–64.

Luengo-Fernandez, R., Leal, J., & Gray, A. 2010. Dementia 2010: *The Prevalence, Economic Cost and Research Funding of Dementia Compared with Other Major Diseases*. Cambridge, England: Alzheimer's Research Trust.

Marshall, M. 2012. *Dementia Friendly Design Guidance for Hospital Wards*. Dementia Services Development Centre. Stirling, Scotland: University of Stirling.

Mast, B. 2014. Whole person assessment and care planning. In *Excellence in Dementia Care*, 2nd edition, edited by Downs, M., & Bowers, B., 290–302. Maidenhead, England: Open University Press.

Moriarty, J., Sharif, N., & Robinson, J. 2011. *Black and Minority Ethnic People with Dementia and Their Access to Support and Services*. London: Social Care Institute for Excellence.

Mukadam, N., Cooper, C., & Livingston, G. 2011. A systematic review of ethnicity and pathways to care in dementia. *International Journal of Geriatric Psychiatry*, 26(1): 12–20.

National Audit Office. 2010. *Improving Dementia Services in England—An Interim Report*. London: TSO.

National Collaborating Centre for Mental Health. 2007—Updated 2011. *Dementia: A NICE-SCIE Guideline on Supporting People with Dementia and Their Carers in Health and Social Care*. National Clinical Practice Guideline Number 42. Leicester, England: British Psychological Society and Gaskell.

NHS England and NHS Improving Quality. 2014. *Dementia Diagnosis and Care in England—Learning from Clinical Commissioning Groups*. Leeds, England: NHS England.

Office for National Statistics. 2012. Population change. In *Pension Trends*, Chapter 2. http://www.ons.gov.uk/ons/search/index.

Prince, M., Bryce, R., & Ferri, C. 2011. *World Alzheimer Report: The Benefits of Early Diagnosis and Intervention*. London: Alzheimer's Disease International.

Royal College of Nursing. 2013. *Dementia: Commitment to the Care of People with Dementia in Hospital Settings*. London: Royal College of Nursing.

Scottish Government. 2013. *Scotland's National Dementia Strategy: 2013–2016*. Edinburgh: Scottish Government.

United Nations. 2011. *Political Declaration of the High-level Meeting of the General Assembly on the Prevention and Control of Non-communicable Diseases*. New York: United Nations.

Welsh Assembly Government. 2011. *National Dementia Vision for Wales*. Cardiff, Wales: Welsh Assembly Government.

Wimo, A. Winbladand, B., & Jonsson, L. 2010. The worldwide societal costs of dementia: Estimates for 2009. *Alzheimer's and Dementia*, 6: 98–105.

Woods, B. 2004. Invited commentary: Non-pharmacological interventions in dementia. *Advances in Psychiatric Treatments*, 10: 178–179.

Woods, L., Smith, G., Pendleton, J., & Parker, D. 2013. *Innovate Dementia Baseline Report: Shaping the Future for People Living with Dementia*. Liverpool, England: Liverpool John Moores University.

World Health Organisation. 2012. *Dementia: A Public Health Priority*. Geneva, Switzerland: World Health Organisation.

Zeisel, J. et al. 2003. Environmental correlates to behavioural health outcomes in Alzheimer's special care units. *The Gerontologist*, 43(5): 697–711.

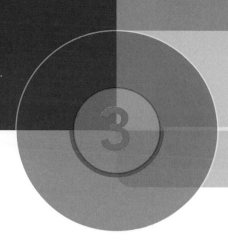

Assessment

DENISE PARKER

AIM

- To consider the importance of the assessment process in a dementia care context

OBJECTIVES

- To identify the role of classifying and diagnosing as part of the early identification of dementia
- To recognise that assessment is a process rather than just a set of tools
- To appreciate that skilful assessment is partnership focused
- To critically reflect on the notion that the assessment process should be holistic

OVERVIEW

Meeting the needs of an aging population is a pressing issue locally, nationally, and globally. As we have greater longevity, the incidences of people experiencing conditions such as dementia will increase (Department of Health [DH], 2009, 2013; Alzheimer's Society, 2014b; Woods et al., 2013). Dementia is a progressive condition that mainly affects older people. It adversely affects cognitive function, behaviour, and the ability to perform daily tasks. It is also viewed as one of the main causes of dependence and disability in older adults (World Health Organisation [WHO], 2003; Alzheimer's Disease International, 2014).

To employ evidence-based strategies to benefit people living with dementia and improve the quality of life for them and their caregivers, practitioners need to have knowledge and understanding of the person's individual lived experience (Woods et al., 2013). This cannot be systematically and professionally constructed without appropriate assessment and comprehensive knowledge of the health and social care system. In addition, the assessment process needs to be sensitive, dignified, and appropriate. It also needs to be timely for it to be most effective (Smith, 2014). Adams (2008) reminded us that assessment is the first part of the nursing process; it is made up of assessment, planning, intervention and evaluation. Indeed, Adams advocated a whole-systems approach to assessment in dementia care and care planning: 'The whole systems approach should shape how dementia care nurses undertake each part of the nursing process, including assessment and care planning' (p. 127).

On this basis the intention of this chapter is to support the development of the learner by providing the opportunity to explore and reflect on the skills and knowledge required to be effective when assessing people living with dementia. It also goes without saying that being effective has a values-based dimension and that it is important for the learner to value and respect the privacy, individuality, dignity and cultural diversity of the person with dementia (Smith, 2014; Alzheimer's Disease International, 2012). To support the learning in this chapter the following scenario is used throughout:

Neville is 62 years old; he lives at home with his partner, David. He has two adult children, Daisy and Robert. Daisy lives in Spain with her husband and two preschool children. Robert's relationship with his father has been strained since he moved in with David 6 years ago, following an acrimonious divorce from his wife and Robert's mother, Diane. He has not visited his father for 6 months, but they do speak on the phone occasionally. His father lives with his wife, Ellie, 2 miles away. Neville has taken early retirement from his job as a primary school teacher, as he felt under pressure to do so due to his perceived and real problems of organising himself and increasing forgetfulness. David is a bus driver and works shifts. The couple enjoy walks with their dog, Max, and grab any time that they can in their touring caravan. They enjoy pub quizzes, particularly at their local pub. They are active members of their community. Neville has been withdrawing more from social events recently and seems quite down in mood. David has attributed this to Neville fretting about his finishing work and his difficult relationship with Robert. However, David has noticed that Neville is quite forgetful and less tolerant to stress these days. Neville himself is defensive about his forgetfulness and his mood. Eventually, David and Daisy persuaded Neville to see his general practitioner (GP).

CLASSIFICATION

Organic disorders come in many types; most people living with organic disorders are not necessarily treated within specialist mental health services. Therefore, it is important the practitioner have an understanding of signs, symptoms and possible treatments (Parker, 2012). Impaired cognitive functioning is the main feature of organic disorders (Parker, 2012). Clinical syndromes like delirium can also be present. Delirium has many causes, including infection (commonly chest or urine infections), high temperature, side effects of medication, sudden withdrawal from drugs or alcohol, liver or kidney dysfunction, brain injury, terminal illness and constipation (Royal College of Psychiatrists, 2009). Psychoactive substances such as alcohol can induce delirium.

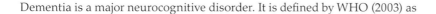

Dementia is a major neurocognitive disorder. It is defined by WHO (2003) as

… a syndrome due to disease of the brain, usually of a chronic disturbance or progressive nature, in which there is of multiple higher cortical functions, including memory, thinking, orientation, comprehension, calculation, learning capacity and judgment. Consciousness is not clouded. The impairments of cognitive function are commonly accompanied, and occasionally preceded, by deterioration in emotional control, social behaviour or motivation. (WHO, 2003: 48)

Dementia tends to be used as an umbrella term which captures a 'group of syndromes characterised by progressive decline in cognition and social functioning, and often associated with increasing age' (Parker, 2012: 123). There is a considerable amount of overlap in the pathology of types of dementia. Peters (2001) suggested that mixed forms of dementia may be more common. Age is the biggest risk factor for having dementia, with up to 31% of older people in hospital and 5% of people living in the community affected by it. People with Down's syndrome have a much greater risk of developing Alzheimer-type dementia, with an earlier onset age of 30 to 40 years old. About 55% of people with Down's syndrome will be affected by dementia at age 60 to 69, as compared with 5% of the remainder of the population. The prevalence of Alzheimer's and other forms of dementia in other people with learning disabilities is no greater than the remainder of the population (DH, 2005).

The National Institute for Health and Clinical Excellence and Social Care Institute for Excellence (NICE/SCIE) (2006) remind us that not everyone with memory problems has dementia; they may have mild cognitive impairment (MCI).

Primary healthcare staff should consider referring people who show signs of mild cognitive impairment (MCI) for assessment by memory assessment services to aid early identification of dementia, because more than 50% of people with MCI later develop dementia. (NICE/SCIE, 2006: 22)

In the UK it was estimated that in 2015 there were 850,000 people diagnosed with dementia, of which 40,000 people were under 65 years of age and 25,000 people were from black and ethnic minority communities. Of these 850,000 people, 677,000 were in England (Alzheimer's Society, 2015c). Diagnosis rates in 2014 were 42.8% for Wales and 64.8% for Northern Ireland (Alzheimer's Society, 2014a). According to the Alzheimer's Society (2015c), of these figures, the diagnosis rates in England were 59%.

It is crucial that we ensure early diagnosis and intervention in dementia care (NICE/SCIE, 2006; DH, 2009; Moniz-Cook & Manthorpe, 2009). We must bear in mind that diagnosis is the start of a journey for the person living with dementia and the person's family. This journey is a difficult one, and we need to empathise with the person newly diagnosed with dementia and those close to them about the impact of such a diagnosis and the fear of the future, whether real or perceived. It is a sobering thought that rates of diagnosis are nowhere near the targets set; however, it is at times a lack of knowledge about dementia that hinders this process (DH, 2009). This was brought to our attention by the Audit Commission (2002), highlighting that only half of GPs saw it as important to actively check for signs of dementia and ascertain an early diagnosis in their patients. Lacking also was clarity of information and psychological support for the person with a diagnosis of dementia and their carers (Audit Commission, 2002).

In 2009, following a long period of anticipation, the strategy documented in *Living Well with Dementia: A National Dementia Strategy* by the Department of Health was published. This document draws on examples of good practice. It covers three key areas: improved awareness, earlier diagnosis and interventions, and a higher quality of care. The strategy has 17 key areas of good practice, including improving public and professional awareness and understanding of dementia and good-quality diagnosis and intervention for all.

However, despite awareness campaigns and reports such as those cited, dementia diagnosis rates are still an issue. Consider what would happen if everyone with dementia were diagnosed: The health and social care system is barely coping now with diagnosis rates unacceptably low (Alzheimer's Society, 2014a; Alzheimer's Society, 2015b). Things are improving following the *Prime Minister's Challenge on Dementia* in 2012 and the followup in 2015 (DH, 2012, 2015) and the national strategy for dementia (DH 2009).

ASSESSMENT AS A PROCESS

Dementia affects different people in different ways, and by its very nature, it does not conform to a clear and sequential pathway (National Collaborating Centre for Mental Health, 2007). Clear assessment that is timely, sensitive, person centred and accurate is crucial. We need to understand the rationale for any assessment used, and we also need to understand when not to use assessment. For example, there may come a point as a person becomes more severely affected in their dementia journey that subjecting them to an assessment such as carrying out a Mini-Mental State Examination (MMSE) just for the sake of doing so verges on cruelty (Folstein, Folstein, & McHugh, 1975). Adams (2008) reminded us that three types of assessment are used in dementia care:

- Assessment of the person with dementia
- Assessment of the family carer(s)
- Assessment of how the person with dementia and their family carer(s) work together

Adams (2008) asserted that assessment of only the person with dementia or the person's carers gives a one-sided view, and a fuller picture is obtained by assessing all three areas. Of course, an assessment is prone to subjectivity and is a snapshot in time, a window into a person's life. Remember that when we look through a window, we do not see the whole view as we are restrained by the window frame. Also, do we see what we want to see and miss some fine or crucial detail? The purpose of the assessment must be kept in mind (it is stressful to be the subject of an assessment); also, the best person in the team to carry out the assessment must be considered. Although the Care Programme Approach (CPA) (DH, 2008) used in specialist mental health services has been around since 1990, we still do not always carry out the process accurately. When considering the CPA process, we see that assessment is only the start of the process, followed by care planning and reviewing, coordinated by a care coordinator. Even in areas where the CPA is not used, the process should be similar: a comprehensive assessment of health and social care needs, with a clear care plan (including risk assessment), coordinated by a key professional. It is this assessment that triggers additional specialist assessments, such as by occupational therapists and speech therapists. Barker (1997) said that nursing assessment focuses on outcomes; although these focuses are important, we also need to acknowledge that the assessment process is an opportunity to find out more about the person with dementia and the person's family.

Information in the assessment process is obtained by various means. This includes the use of semistructured interviews, which are exploratory, giving people with dementia and their carers time to tell their stories (Smith, 2014; Parker, 2012). By using specific questionnaires and rating scales which focus on eliciting specific information (Smith, 2014), these types of assessment methods are used in areas such as memory clinics and by specialists, and an extensive range of tests might be used. Another method is through direct observation; the health and social care practitioner observes and reports information about the service user's behaviours. Generally the practitioner will use all these types of assessment approaches to ensure collecting as much information as possible (Smith, 2014).

To assist the practitioner in understanding cognitive assessment the Alzheimer's Society (2015a) produced a toolkit. According to this, 'measuring someone's cognitive function is one of the most important assessments clinicians make, particularly those in old age psychiatry and geriatric medicine—It is key to detecting dementia and delirium' (p. 3).

Next, we return to the scenario:

Neville's confusion worsened when he had a chest infection, He was given antibiotics, and the confusion subsided to a noticeable extent. However, when they visited Dr Ahmed, David told him that he had concerns that things were not 'normal', and that Neville had not been himself for quite a while. During the consultation, they mentioned how things had been in recent months. For example, Neville had been more irritable than usual and easily distracted and frustrated. At times, he did not really know why. He agreed that he feels as if his mind is not clear and feels a bit like 'a sieve'. David said that he has noticed that Neville's renowned sense of humour is not what it was. Neville now often takes things the wrong way, whereas before he may have laughed. David now feels that he is 'walking on eggshells' at times. Occasionally, he explained, he has seen Neville standing in the kitchen looking bewildered, such as when making meals that he easily tackled previously. This could be due to a lack of concentration. The low point was when Neville served up a half-cooked chicken and became angry when David would not eat it. An argument ensued. This seems to be a daily event, and both partners are left feeling drained and angry. However, David is wondering if something is seriously wrong. He just wants Neville back to normal.

Neville's condition was reviewed by his GP following the CQUIN (Commissioning for Quality and Innovation) target for dementia (NHS England, 2014). This meant that the payment given to the practice by the National Health Service (NHS) was dependent on targets being met, in this case screening for dementia being carried out. The CQUIN target for dementia and delirium has four elements regarding people with dementia in the hospital: find, assess, investigate and refer (p. 32). Also, the GP was dementia aware. Over recent years, awareness of dementia had been improved amongst the practice staff (Audit Commission, 2002; DH, 2001, 2009, 2012, 2015; NHS England, 2014). The GP considered that Neville's difficulties with cognition and everyday life could be due to MCI or indeed to dementia (NICE/SCIE, 2006; WHO, 2003).

SKILLFUL ASSESSMENT

Smith (2014) noted that assessment is a fundamental part of mental health nursing practice; however, of course, it is fundamental to any practitioner's practice. Smith (2014) notes that assessment is driven by the therapeutic relationship and should be person centred, collaborative, and underpinned by effective communication skills.

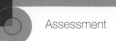

> Just take some time and imagine how Neville in the scenario must have felt being assessed.

In the mid-1990s, the author worked at a development post using action research (Williamson, Bellman, & Webster, 2011) to integrate the CPA and care management. At the start of the project the author had to ascertain assessments used by the different disciplines in the multidisciplinary team. It was quickly realised that assessment was not an exact science, and that assessment tools and assessment skills varied widely. One person mentioned not carrying a paper assessment, with the assessment all in the person's head. This anecdote raises a serious point: Assessment is prone to subjectivity although it does rely on advanced communication skills of observation, questioning, active listening, empathy, clarifying and the ability to summarise (O'Carroll & Park, 2007; Smith, 2014). Also, those skills include the abilities to both record information with accuracy and interpret the information effectively. Adams (2008) commented that there is likely to be a degree of subjectivity in all nursing assessments because practitioners are not there to merely gather the facts. In addition, practitioners have to be skilled in deciding how best to represent different versions of events. One way of doing this according to Tanner and Harris (2008) is to develop a person-centred approach to assessment.

Of course, practitioners are required to know the evidence base and rationale for any assessment tools used; along with assessment skills, practitioners also have to be able to develop a care plan, evaluate care, and coordinate. A skill following assessment is to ascertain with the person with dementia and the person's carers (professional and informal carers) the interventions required. According to Moniz-Cook and Manthorpe (2009), when psychosocial interventions are selected to aid the person with dementia or their carers, as practitioners we need to consider a number of issues. Initially, the person's situation and wishes need exploring. Choosing relevant interventions requires a focussed assessment which integrates the personal profile, biography, the person's relationships, motivations and areas of interest, as well as family and other support. This could be jointly done, or by self-assessment. The practitioner then needs to look at how to arrange and plan the best support to offer; this includes supporting the carer. Let us consider the carer's role from a personal perspective:

As a registered carer myself for a close relative living with dementia (mixed vascular and Alzheimer's), the role, along with a full-time, demanding job and other commitments, can at times feel overwhelming, and I am a registered mental health nurse who specialises in dementia care. I constantly ask myself: 'How would I cope without knowing what I know and having the skills that I have?' On the other hand, I sometimes wonder if the opposite is the question that I should be asking. That is, am I hindered by my knowledge and professional values and baggage? My personal and professional personas are entwined, and I cannot ignore either. Perhaps I reflect too much. Hence, on writing here on the subject of carer assessment, I am wearing two hats, one of carer and one of professional. I have personally experienced, as a carer, being assessed. It is not all negative. I have learnt a lot from this role; yes, it is a hard job, but there are rewards also. I have seen glimpses of my relative from the past, of memories of good times, of times that I was privy to, and of a world hitherto hidden to me, for example, related to personhood, childhood and 'being'. I see glimpses into my relative's childhood and pieces of jigsaws to make me understand my relative better. I am forced to give of myself the most precious gift that I can give (but at the same time, it feels resented by me at times, such as at 11 p.m. at night, when I have to go home to be up for work at 6 a.m.)—this gift is time and love. We laugh, we have fun.

I am a better person for it. But, I do not know of an assessment that picks up this richness, quirkiness, and multifaceted aspects of myself, my relative, and other family members who are also carers the same as I am. I am one of six siblings, and if participating in a carer assessment, I can guarantee that none of the assessments would be the same. For sure, one thing is the same: We all have our relative's best interests at heart, want the best. However, I know that for each of the six of us, this is not homogeneous.

Added to the mix mentioned, different agencies and people have their own views of what is happening in caring for people with dementia. According to Adams (2008), nursing assessments need to capture these views, allowing various people to have a say and state fully what has happened, what is happening, and what needs to happen. (This can be said for assessments carried out by all practitioners.) Of course, we sometimes lose sight that at the centre of it all is the person living with dementia.

HOLISTIC ASSESSMENT

Person-centred assessment has become more of the norm in health and social care, and as such is still in danger of becoming a paper exercise and taken for granted. Mast (2014: 291) stated that 'The person centred approach argues that people with dementia are more than the sum of their cognitive and functional impairments.' Kitwood (1997) and others stress that people with dementia deserve to be respected, valued and honoured, the key attributes of personhood. Mast (2014) suggested that although understanding the nature of functional and cognitive impairments is important, we need to realise that there is a lot more that we need to understand about the person to optimize their experience of living with dementia, enhance quality of life, and reduce excess disability. To do so the whole person needs assessment (holistic assessment) of the following (Mast, 2014):

- The dementia, including cognitive and functional changes
- The person, including their likes, wants, needs, and aspirations
- The person's experience of dementia and how life has changed

The person with dementia may also have other co-morbid conditions that have to be addressed at the same time. Co-morbid conditions can include physical conditions such as diabetes and hypertension or mental health conditions such as depression and anxiety (Alzheimer's Disease International, 2014).

In addition to and building on Kitwood's (1997) 'malignant social psychology' notion the practitioner has to consider it is not only the effects of the disease process of dementia on the person that causes a deterioration of functioning and cognitive decline, but also the negative impact of professional and family carers disempowering and disenfranchising the person under the auspices of 'care'. Nichols et al. (1998) found that 39% of people in their study of nursing home residents (177 incontinent residents in four venues) diagnosed with dementia made consistent decisions that compared with peers who did not have dementia. This shows that people with dementia in certain circumstances can have significant capacity to make health-care decisions. Of course, we have the Equality Act (2010) and the Mental Capacity Act (2005) to compel the practitioner to consider issues of capacity, inclusion and diversity (Equality Act, 2010; Mental Capacity Act, 2005).

The practitioner must not lose sight of the 'personhood' (Kitwood, 1997) of the person living with dementia, always see the person as an individual, and realise the fact that middle-aged and older people have a lifetime of coping with life events. The context for each person needs to be given attention; for example, the 'baby boomers' (the postwar generation born between the late 1940s until 1963) are now entering the 'older adult' age group. They may be too young to remember or have lived through life without the welfare state and the NHS. Their lifestyle and expectations may be different from those of individuals born a generation earlier. 'Older people' are not to be seem as a homogeneous group. They are more likely than younger people to have been bereaved of a near relation, partner or child or to have a debilitating physical or life-limiting condition. Other loss issues could be due to the aging process itself, a result of living in a society that values youth. An older person may have invested self-worth in a youthful self-image. When this is threatened or compromised, self-esteem may be affected. Loss may be experienced on multiple levels: youth, loss of significant others, either by bereavement or literally by geographical distance, employment, and their perceptions of usefulness and lifestyle (Parker, 2012).

Assessing holistically can be time consuming and it can be easy, during a busy day and in a busy job which is often task orientated, for assessment to become a process of filling in a form, and for the assessment to become a 'dry' document. However, the practitioner needs to keep in mind how hugely stressful it is for any of us to be assessed or, put another way, examined or scrutinised. An assessment is meant to be a 'living' document and should reflect the life and experiences of the person living with dementia. The assessment process is also the cornerstone of making decisions which are based on information that has been collected; it assists the practitioner in making sense of the person with dementia and their situation (Barker, 1997; Smith, 2014). As a questioning process it should promote curiosity within the practitioner, creating a desire to know more about what and who they are assessing and why, and ultimately considering whether the assessment process is fit for purpose (Taylor & White, 2000).

Returning to Neville and thinking critically within a holistic context:

- Neville has hypertension and is on medication. Is his blood pressure being monitored by the practice nurse?
- Neville is exhibiting signs of lowness in mood. Is he feeling depressed, and has he been assessed for depression?
- Neville is at times confused. Did the GP assess for signs of delirium?

CHAPTER SUMMARY

Meeting the needs of an aging population is a pressing issue. It is also a challenge. With greater longevity of the population the incidence of people living with dementia will increase. Dementia is a progressive condition and it is one of the main causes of dependence and disability in older adults. To provide the best quality care for people living with dementia practitioners need to have good knowledge and understanding of the person's individual lived experience.

Dementia as a major neurocognitive disorder can come in different types and present in different ways, especially if other conditions may be present, such as delirium. On this basis the practitioner has to have good understanding of signs, symptoms and treatments. Ensuring that people receive an early diagnosis of dementia is an ongoing challenge that is continually addressed through a number of strategies and policies.

As dementia affects different people in different ways, it is important that the assessment process is timely, sensitive, person centred and accurate. Three types of assessment are used in dementia care; using all three will ensure a fuller picture of the person's needs and circumstances. Assessment is a fundamental part of the health and social care practitioner's practice.

It is driven by the therapeutic relationship and should be person centred and collaborative, and underpinned by effective communication skills.

The assessment process should be truly person centred and not just a paper exercise; it should respect, value and honour the person with dementia. The whole person needs assessing which includes understanding the person's experience of dementia and how the person's life has changed.

REFLECTION ON LEARNING

1. Assessment is the first part of the nursing process. Describe the other parts.
2. As a progressive condition, what does dementia adversely affect?
3. Delirium has many causes. What do these include?
4. What does the term *dementia* define?
5. Describe the three types of assessment that are used in dementia care.
6. What does the abbreviation CPA stand for?
7. What should drive the assessment process?
8. Describe the advanced communication skills on which the assessment process relies.
9. What does the person-centred approach argue?
10. What is Kitwood's (1997) notion?

REFERENCES

Adams, T. 2008. *Dementia Care Nursing: Promoting Well-Being in People with Dementia and Their Families*. Basingstoke, UK: Palgrave MacMillan.

Alzheimer's Disease International. 2012. *Overcoming the Stigma of Dementia*. London: Alzheimer's Disease International.

Alzheimer's Disease International. 2014. *World Alzheimer Report 2014: Dementia and Risk Reduction—An Analysis of Protective and Modifiable Factors*. London: Alzheimer's Disease International.

Alzheimer's Society. 2014a. Dementia Diagnosis Rates. http://www.alzheimers.org.uk/site/scripts/documents_info.php?documentID=2165.

Alzheimer's Society. 2014b. *Dementia 2014: Opportunity for Change*. London: Alzheimer's Society.

Alzheimer's Society. 2015a. *Helping You to Assess Cognition: A Practical Toolkit for Clinicians*. London: Alzheimer's Society.

Alzheimer's Society. 2015b. Right to Know Campaign Diagnosis and Support. http://www.alzheimers.org.uk/site/scripts/documents_info.php?documentID=1521&pageNumber=2.

Alzheimer's Society. 2015c. Statistics. http://www.alzheimers.org.uk/statistics.

Audit Commission. 2002. *Forget Me Not 2002: Developing Mental Health Services for Older People*. London: Audit Commission.

Barker, P. 1997. *Assessment in Psychiatric and Mental Health Nursing: In Research of the Whole Person*. Cheltenham, UK: Thornes.

Department of Health. 2001. *The National Service Framework for Older People*. London: Department of Health.

Department of Health. 2008. *Refocusing the Care Programme Approach: Policy and Positive Practice Guidance*. London: Department of Health.

Department of Health. 2009. *Living Well with Dementia: A National Dementia Strategy.* London: Department of Health.

Department of Health. 2012. *Prime Minister's Challenge on Dementia: Delivering Major Improvements in Dementia Care and Research by 2015.* London: Department of Health.

Department of Health. 2013. *Dementia: A State of the Nation Report on Dementia Care and Support in England.* London: Department of Health.

Department of Health. 2015. *Prime Minister's Challenge on Dementia 2020.* London: Department of Health.

Equality Act. 2010. http://www.legislation.gov.uk/ukpga/2010/15/contents.

Folstein, M., Folstein, S.E., & McHugh, P.R. 1975. 'Mini Mental State': A practical method for grading the cognitive state of patients for the clinician. *Journal of Psychiatric Research,* 12(3): 189–198.

Kitwood, T. 1997. *Dementia Reconsidered.* London: Open University Press.

Mast, B. 2014. Whole person assessment and care planning. In *Excellence in Dementia Care,* 2nd edition, edited by Downs, M., & Bowers, B., 290–302. Maidenhead, UK: Open University Press.

Mental Capacity Act. 2005. http://www.legislation.gov.uk/ukpga/2005/9/contents.

Moniz-Cook, E., & Manthorpe, J. (Editors). 2009. *Early Psychological Interventions in Dementia: Evidence-Based Practice.* London: Kingsley.

National Collaborating Centre for Mental Health. 2007—Updated 2011. *Dementia: A NICE-SCIE Guideline on Supporting People with Dementia and Their Carers in Health and Social Care.* National Clinical Practice Guideline Number 42. Leicester, UK: British Psychological Society and Gaskell.

National Institute for Health and Clinical Excellence and Social Care Institute for Excellence. 2006. *Dementia: Supporting People with Dementia and Their Carers in Health and Social Care.* NICE Clinical Guideline 42. London: NICE & SCIE.

NHS England. 2014. *Commissioning for Quality and Innovation (CQUIN) 2014/15 Guidance.* London: NHS Commissioning Board.

Nichols, J., Phillips, M., Belisle, S., Sansone, P., & Scmitt, L. 1998. Determining the capacity of demented nursing home residents to name a health care proxy. *Clinical Gerontologist,* 19: 35–50.

O'Carroll, M., & Park, A. 2007. *Essential Mental Health Nursing Skills.* London: Mosby.

Parker, D. 2012. Psychological interventions and working with the older adult. In *Psychological Interventions,* edited by Smith, G., 120–132. Maidenhead, UK: Open University Press.

Peters, R. 2001. The prevention of dementia. *Journal of Cardiovascular Risk,* 8: 253–256.

Royal College of Psychiatrists. 2009. *Factsheet: Delirium.* London: Royal College of Psychiatrists.

Smith, G. 2014. *Mental Health Nursing at a Glance.* Chichester, UK: Wiley Blackwell.

Tanner, D., & Harris, J. 2008. *Working with Older People.* Abingdon, UK: Routledge.

Taylor, C., & White, C. 2000. *Practising Reflexivity in Health and Welfare: Making Knowledge.* Buckingham, UK: Open University Press.

Williamson, G.R., Bellman, L., & Webster, J. 2011. *Action Research in Nursing and Healthcare.* London: Sage.

Woods, L., Smith, G., Pendleton, J., & Parker, D. 2013. *Innovate Dementia Baseline Report: Shaping the Future for People Living with Dementia.* Liverpool, UK: Liverpool John Moores University.

World Health Organisation. 2003. *International Statistical Classification of Diseases and Related Health Problems.* 10th revision. Geneva, Switzerland: WHO.

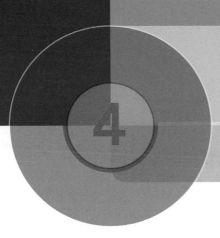

Case management

DENISE PARKER

AIM

- To consider the importance of the case management process within a dementia care context

OBJECTIVES

- To define case management
- To identify the different case management models
- To appreciate assessment within a case-finding context
- To recognise the role of care planning and its core components

OVERVIEW

This chapter explores case management and dementia care. Two case studies are used to illustrate challenges faced by individuals living with dementia and their families: the cases of Annie and Beryl and their caregivers. However, it is evident that there is not a common, agreed definition of case management (Koch et al., 2012). This, therefore, makes it difficult to use it as a basis for commentary and research. Essentially case management consists of four components: assessment, care planning, review, and a case manager. Besides the issue of endeavouring to achieve early diagnosis of people living with dementia, it follows that intervention following diagnosis is essential (National Collaborating Centre for Mental Health, 2007; Department of Health [DH], 2009, 2012, 2013, 2015; Moniz-Cook & Manthorpe, 2009). Although diagnosis is the start of a journey for the person living with dementia and their family, the journey for the person with dementia and their caregivers subsequently follows a pathway that can be seemingly straightforward from the start of the journey for some people. The National Dementia Strategy (DH, 2009) aspires that every person diagnosed with dementia will have access to a support worker who is a care navigator to help them navigate their way through the support system.

Inevitably, the person's needs become more complex as the disease process takes its course, frequently co-existing with possible complications of other long-term or acute health conditions and frailty. This means that eventually a large proportion of people will be subject to the case management process, even for a short period of time, to prevent hospitalisation or further hospitalisation. To add to the mix of complexity, we have to consider that diagnosis rates of dementia are not at their optimum level in the UK and globally. Also, health-care systems such as in the UK and Northern Europe are having to confront the reality that there is not yet a cure for dementia and are concentrating more on improving quality of life for people living with dementia by looking at such areas as psychosocial interventions, exercise, lighting and nutrition, for example, as extolled by the European Innovate Dementia Project (Woods et al., 2013; DH, 2010).

Alzheimer's Disease International (in conceding that dementia is an epidemic on a global scale) states that 'the number of people living with dementia worldwide today is estimated at 44 million, set to almost double by 2030 and more than triple by 2050. The global cost of dementia was estimated in 2010 at US$604 billion, and this is only set to rise' (2014: 1). The report further states that governments must develop strategies to ensure that the dementia 'epidemic' is tackled holistically, by reducing risk factors and caring adequately for people living with dementia and supporting their families and friends. However, should everyone with dementia be identified and diagnosed, the probability is that few nations, if any, would be able to properly and adequately meet their needs.

The need to rationalise and strategically target resources in health and social care has always been present, but the pressure has been felt more in recent years due to the global recession. Case management is a way of finding and focusing on those individuals deemed most in need of it, by virtue of the levels of risk, complexity, and older age, particularly those living with dementia. The aim is to minimise risk and to enable these individuals to live in the community longer. One of the main aims of the *Living Well with Dementia: A National Dementia Strategy'* (DH, 2009) document was to improve care for people living with dementia at every part of their journey, from diagnosis onwards.

DEFINING CASE MANAGEMENT

Dementia is a CQUIN (Commissioning for Quality and Innovation) target (NHS England, 2014); the goal is

> … to incentivise the identification of patients with dementia and delirium, alone, and in combination alongside their other medical conditions, to prompt appropriate referral and follow up after they leave hospital and to ensure that hospitals deliver high quality care to people with dementia and support their carers. (p. 29)

Koch et al. (2012) considered the potential of case management for people with dementia. They carried out a critical comparison of identified studies in two systematic reviews of case management trials in dementia care, with selective inclusion of studies that were nontrial and economic evaluations. This led them to provisionally conclude that firstly, studies with long periods of follow-up indicated delayed admission to care homes for people living with dementia. Secondly, the chances of relocation may be influenced by the quality of life of people with dementia and their carers. Thirdly, due to differing understandings of what case management is, it is difficult to interpret studies. Fourthly, Koch et al. were in agreement that the population who would benefit most from case management requires characterisation.

Case management was rolled out as part of the UK government introduction of community matrons (DH 2004). In the UK, the community matron was a new specialist role to support people with long-term complex conditions. There is no common consensus of what "case management" consists of (Koch et al., 2012; Ross, Curry, & Goodwin, 2011). It is a generically used term, with multiple definitions. Essentially, it is the process of planning, coordinating and reviewing a person's care, with the broad aim of improving the person's quality of life in a cost-effective and efficient manner (Hutt, Rosen, & McCauley, 2004). Hutt, Rosen, and McCauley (2004) state:

> There is no single model of case management, and the term is used to provide a range of approaches to improve the organisation and co-ordination of services for people with severe, and complex health problems. … The core elements of case management are case finding, or screening, assessment, care planning, implementation, monitoring and review. They may be undertaken as the specific job of a 'case manager' or as a series of tasks fulfilled by members of a team. (p. 1)

Boaden et al. (2006: i) described case management as follows:

> Case management for frail elderly people aims to combine both preventive and responsive care for patients at high risk of deterioration in their health.

It includes

- Defining a target group of patients
- Individual assessment and care planning
- Monitoring of patients on a regular basis and intervening when problems arise

CASE MANAGEMENT MODELS

A plethora of case management models exists in the National Health Service (NHS). Some examples are:

Guided Care. A model for use with individuals experiencing chronic disease. It originated in 2001 in the United States. A specially trained and highly skilled registered nurse works in primary care with three to four doctors, providing high-quality care to patients with chronic conditions (seven or more conditions). Predictive modelling software is used, analysing risk and probability of hospitalisation based on the individual's profile in the past year. Care is managed in primary care, with the Guided Care nurse carrying out an assessment of the person and the person's carer at home (Boult, Karm, & Groves, 2008; Ross, Curry, & Goodwin, 2011; Wolff et al., 2011).

PACE (Program of All-Inclusive Care for the Elderly). This is a US programme with the intent of maintaining frail older adults over the age of 55 at home longer. It is an integrated model of care that has been in existence for over 30 years. Those eligible for PACE are considered by the state to require long-term nursing home care. The PACE case management model provides care in day centres via multidisciplinary teams. The team shares accountability and allocates resources. This is facilitated by a data system which gathers data on all aspects of the individual's health, thus forming the basis of the care plan. Health and social care resources are integrated (Ross, Curry, & Goodwin, 2011; Curry & Ham, 2010; International Value Cases, 2013).

Virtual wards. This model of case management was developed in the UK and is widely utilised by the NHS. Although the form of the model can vary, the premise is that it is based on the concept of a hospital ward, which is replicated in the community. There are 'virtual' ward rounds, and patients' needs are reviewed depending on risk. Review could be daily, weekly, or monthly. There is a multidisciplinary team and a ward clerk. The ward clerk is the main point of contact. An early intervention approach is used, as is a predictive risk model. Patients deemed to have the highest risk are admitted to the virtual ward. The case manager is a general practitioner (GP) or a community matron; evaluation indicates positive levels of patient satisfaction and reduction in hospital admissions (Ross, Curry, & Goodwin, 2011; Ham & Oldham, 2009; Lewis et al., 2013).

CPA (Care Programme Approach; used in specialist mental health care, including dementia care). This model of case management was introduced in 1991 by the NHS. It is a model for assessment, care planning, care coordination and review of people diagnosed with mental health conditions and complex needs. This includes people experiencing dementia. Central to the process of CPA is the involvement of service users and their caregivers. A care coordinator is the lynchpin of the care package and oversees the care plan, ensures that reviews happen, and is the main point of contact for the person (DH, 2008).

Single assessment process. The National Service Framework for Older People (DH, 2001) set out the concept of a single assessment process for older people to avoid duplication and so the people received a timely, appropriate and effective response to meet their needs (Abendstern et al., 2010). A single assessment process meant that there would be one set of documentation that all disciplines involved in the person's care would use. However, although this process was envisaged, disappointingly, it has not gathered real momentum and taken root.

Evercare case management model (derived from the United States). This model gave frail older adults and their carers extra contacts, monitoring and options for treatment. However, in an evaluation by Boaden et al. (2006), this model did not make an impact on reducing hospital admissions, but it did make a positive impact on quality-of-life issues and patient satisfaction. The evaluation involved a pilot study of nine Primary Care Trusts (PCTs) in the UK. Patients and carers reported satisfaction, particularly concerning the role of the main practitioner involved (advanced primary nurse), including for psychological support, medication monitoring, rapid crisis response, advocacy, and education and information about the patient's condition. As time passed, general practitioners took more of a back seat in the patient's direct care. They acted also in a supervisory capacity to the advanced primary nurses.

Consider the family dynamics that might unfold during Annie's dementia journey and how this may have an impact on case management:

Annie O'Brien was an 84-year-old widow who lived in a small town in the north of England. She lived in a housing trust bungalow in a corner of a large social housing estate. She had lived on the same estate (but not always in the bungalow) for 44 years. She had a large family of four daughters and two sons. She was in the fortunate situation that all of her daughters lived in the same town. She had been a widow for 15 years. She missed John, her husband. She had 20 grandchildren, all grown, and 17 great-grandchildren (the eldest was 15). Annie could be described as a 'matriarch' and had always had a strong and domineering demeanour toward her children, peppered with a capacity for great kindness and generosity. Subsequently, some of her children had relied on her for advice (good or bad) and most of the children for borrowing money. She always threatened her children that they must never put her in a home and implied that it was their duty to look after her in old age as she 'reared them'. She was religious, and the commandment 'Honour thy father and thy mother' was amongst many quotations that were often given by both parents to the children as mantras during their formative years. Hell was the place that they would go to if they did not follow the Ten Commandments. Also, as Annie was growing up, it was not the cultural norm for elders to be in care unless it was the workhouse. She had heard tales of the workhouse from her older relatives. In Annie's psyche, this translated to residential and nursing care homes, although she had little experience of visiting people in them. She compelled her children to promise her that they would never put her in a home. Her own parents and parents-in-law had died before old age, when she was a young woman. Therefore, she had never experienced caring for an aged parent or grandparent. She did not believe in mental illness, which she saw as a weakness. She passed these views on to most of her children. Although she was one of eight siblings, Annie was the last surviving sibling. She was close to them, even though they argued often and would not speak for long periods at a time. Over the last 3 years, she had many losses of family, friends, neighbours and her pet dog. As her social circle dwindled, and as she had poor mobility, her main social contacts were with her children. She went to church regularly with two of them. Dynamics of kinship, loyalty, guilt and duty were at play here. After arguments and accusations directed at Joan, Annie's daughter who broached the subject that Annie may have dementia, it was agreed that Annie would go to the GP with a couple of her children. Most of the children had denied that there was even a problem, despite much evidence to the contrary. Annie was diagnosed with vascular dementia at the age of 81. In some ways, this was the start of a journey of discovery, facing reality and continuing denial by Annie herself and most of her family.

Annie continued to live at home alone. Her mobility was poor. Despite members of the care team and family members asking her to consider removing her rugs, she refused. Although there was an issue of her being deemed to lack mental capacity (Mental Capacity Act, 2005), she defined a home as having a hearth rug. One night, she tripped over it. She cut her head on the fireplace and fractured her hip. She had a falls monitor at the time, and staff from the telecare call centre contacted her daughter. The community wardens came to the house and called paramedics. Annie was confused and scared. She was admitted to the local hospital and underwent a hip replacement. The clinical team liaised with the community multidisciplinary team, including her GP, who had been caring for Annie. It was agreed that Annie could no longer go on living alone at home. Eventually, the family agreed with this decision. When Annie was discharged initially, she went into a generic residential home for older people. Following a chest infection, which led to further hospitalisation, the residential home would not take Annie back. They said that

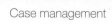

her needs were too complex. Again, Annie had to endure the disruption of a change of accommodation. By this time, she was confused, frail, and near the end of her life. She passed away a year later.

The following is Beryl's story:

Beryl Davenport is 79 years old. She lives a mile away from Annie O'Brien. She has two daughters, one of whom lives nearby. She has one grandson who lives in France. Beryl is independent and does not want to be dependent on her family in her old age. She set up a lasting power of attorney for both finance and health decisions in the event that she loses mental capacity (Mental Capacity Act, 2005). She was a carer for her mother, who experienced dementia in the 1970s and 1980s. Her mother lived her last years in a large psychiatric hospital. Beryl felt that she had no control over decisions made about her mother. It was not the norm for people institutionalised with dementia, or indeed their carers, to be involved in decisions about their care. The attitude was that nothing could be done, and that dementia (or senile dementia, as it was called then) was a 'living death'. Over the years, Beryl has taken an interest in dementia care. She asked her daughters 'what if it happens to me?' Beryl has noticed that she is forgetting details of conversations and missing appointments. She has become reliant on her diary. She panicked at the thought that she may have dementia and may end up like her mother, institutionalised and 'speaking gibberish'. Although embarrassed, she asked her friend Alwyn to come to the GP with her. She was referred to a memory clinic, where she was given a diagnosis of Alzheimer's disease. She asked her daughters to come for dinner and broke the news to them. After their initial upset, Beryl led from the front. She told them that she did not want to be treated any differently, but that she would value their support. As a family, they looked into what dementia was and took up the offer of going to a postdiagnostic group set up by the clinical team for people experiencing dementia and their carers.

ASSESSMENT

Case finding is the first stage of case management: Individuals are identified to be case managed. The aim of this is to prevent people with long-term conditions or frail older people with several conditions being admitted to hospital by supporting them more in the community. It is an essential part of the case management process. Such individuals are deemed to be at high risk of hospitalisation. According to Ross et al. (2011), using case-finding techniques maximises cost effectiveness. Cummings et al. (1997) suggest that across any population, a small number of individuals use the most resources. This means that those people most at risk need to be targeted. Returning to Beryl's story:

Beryl was not identified as suitable for case management. She had made provision for her future by registering the lasting power of attorney so that her daughter would eventually make decisions on her behalf, and Beryl had made an advanced directive (Mental Capacity

Act, 2005). Beryl and her daughter fully engaged with services. Beryl had decided to go into an 'Extra Care' accommodation (housing for people usually over the age of 55, with support that increases as the person's needs become more complex). Beryl was supported by a care navigator (DH, 2009) following her and her daughter attending a postdiagnostic group on being diagnosed with dementia. She was supported by a clinical team, with her main contact a community mental health nurse.

Although in Dutton's (2009) review of the literature from 1998 to 2008 of Extra Care housing and people with dementia, there was no strong evidence base and a lack of rigour in the research, with very few studies focussing on the characteristics, experiences and outcomes of residents with dementia, Dutton did identify important outcomes for people with dementia in Extra Care housing (pp. 101–102):

- Maximisation of dignity and independence
- Individualised activities and experiences that bring pleasure and a sense of accomplishment
- Effective communication
- Meaningful social interactions
- Ability to maintain meaningful relationships
- Person-centred care
- Freedom from pain and discomfort
- The ability to age in place
- The appropriateness, layout and appearance of the physical environment
- Access to health care and palliative care when needed.

The following returns to the case of Annie:

Annie would not consider a lasting power of attorney when she was first diagnosed with dementia. Her family members were offered the chance to go to a postdiagnostic group and they did not take up the offer. This was partly because the members who would have liked to attend with their mother worked, and those who were able to go did not see its relevance. Its usefulness was never really explained to them by the clinical team. As time went on and Annie's condition became more complex and she became more frail, she was deemed to be a candidate for case management. Annie was subject to the CPA, the specialist case management system used in mental health services (DH, 2008, 2011).

In the assessment process involving people living with dementia, there is a chance that those caring for them will focus mainly on cognition and functioning. The case management process compels us to use a more holistic approach to assessment. Mast (2014) mentioned 'whole person assessment' (p. 298), in which the assessment highlights the opportunity to emphasise current and past chapters in the person's life and to link them to how the remaining chapters could be written, thus optimising the person to live the best life possible. After the person is deemed suitable for case management using the case-finding process, assessment needs to relate to the person's current level of functioning and health and social care needs (Ross, Curry, & Goodwin, 2011). The fact that persons are subject to case management means that their needs are complex. The package of care that is thought to be appropriate to the person's needs (this should be in consultation with the person) is dependent on the outcome of the assessment. The health and well-being of the carer also need to be taken into account (DH, 2009; Adams, 2008).

CARE PLANNING

The aim of care planning is to co-create a plan which the individual understands and is in agreement with. When working with people living with dementia, there may be issues of mental capacity (Mental Capacity Act, 2005), but even when the person lacks mental capacity, the plan needs to be made in line with the person's values and preferences and involvement in the process. Mast (2014) argues that when working with people living with dementia, it is not always straightforward to ascertain what an individual wants and then to make it happen, and that there will always be a tension between risk management and the wish to meet the person's needs and respect their values. Mast also states that in care planning, even when the person is no longer able to make personal decisions, the aim is to create the plan with an understanding of the person and their preferences, but with an appreciation of the influence the dementia-related changes may have on how those preferences are met.

As with the notion of whole-person assessment mentioned by Mast (2014), 'whole person care planning' (p. 298), which is influenced by a wider understanding of the person, is also mentioned. The aim is to keep as much continuity as possible, despite the considerable level of change. The care plan is co-created with the person living with dementia, informed by their ability level and preferences. Interventions in the care package need to enhance the person's sense of well-being and 'self' and be in line with current evidence (Parker, 2012).

Central to successful care planning is the competency of the case coordinator to carry out the task. In the care of specialist mental health case management, it is more likely that the case manager will be known as a 'care coordinator' under the CPA (DH, 2008). This is the case in mainstream dementia services for individuals with complex needs. According to Ross et al. (2011), case management has most effectiveness when it is part of a programme approach, working alongside other strategies aimed at supporting more integration and coordination for those individuals with long-term conditions.

The case manager (or in the CPA [DH, 2008], care coordinator) has the pivotal role of ensuring that the process of case management runs smoothly. A good case manager requires many skills; these include the following:

- Accountability
- An understanding of roles and remits of other professionals and agencies
- Excellent communication and interpersonal skills
- Problem-solving skills
- Negotiation and advocacy skills
- An understanding of interventions
- Good assessment skills
- Ability to manage a caseload
- Ability to reflect

Case coordination is a dynamic, moving process. It is necessary for professionals to see the documentation as 'live' documents and the process as ongoing. In fact, each interaction with the person with dementia and the person's carer is a 'review', albeit not always a formal one. If we do not see it as such, then we are doing the individual, their carers, and our colleagues a disservice. Boult et al. (2008) state, in writing about the Guided Care model, that monitoring is proactive. Monitoring and review can take on various forms, such as by a formal meeting or by telephone interview. The reasons for case closure in case management are varied. Models are meant to be ongoing or time limited. Any model of case management aspires to enable the person to self-manage care, often with the support of family carers (Phillips et al., 2014). In the case of people living with dementia, discharge from case management is often due to relocation to a care facility or death.

CHAPTER SUMMARY

Diagnosis is the start of a journey for the person living with dementia and their family; this journey should follow a straightforward pathway with assistance given through a care navigator. Case management is part of this process; essentially it consists of four components: assessment, care planning, review, and a case manager.

Case management forms part of the community matrons initiative. There is no common consensus of what case management is, however it is a process by which care is planned, coordinated, and reviewed with a focus on improving the quality of life of service users and their carers in a cost-effective and efficient manner.

Case finding is part of the assessment process and is the first stage of case management. It aims to prevent people with long term conditions including dementia from being unnecessarily admitted to hospital. People at risk of hospitalisation are identified and community-based services are provided as required.

Care planning is a partnership-orientated process which takes into account a person's values and preferences. It should be holistic and influenced by a wider understanding of the person. Planned interventions need to enhance the person's sense of well-being and self and be evidence based. This process should be led by a case coordinator, who should have the skills to ensure the process is effective and runs smoothly. The care-planning process should be monitored and reviewed and where required the care plan should be amended accordingly to ensure a person's needs are being fully met.

REFLECTION ON LEARNING

1. What should follow diagnosis?
2. What is one of the main aims of the *Living Well with Dementia: A National Dementia Strategy* (DH, 2009) document?
3. What is the goal of dementia as a CQUIN target?
4. What are the core elements of case management?
5. What does PACE as an acronym mean?
6. When was CPA (Care Programme Approach) first introduced?
7. When assessing, what does case management compel practitioners to use?
8. Whose health and well-being also needs to be taken into account during the assessment process?
9. What is the aim of care planning?
10. What is central to successful care planning?

REFERENCES

Abendstern, M., Hughes, J., Clarkson, P., Sutcliffe, C., Wilson, K., & Challis, D. 2010. 'We need to talk': communication between primary care and other health and social care agencies following the introduction of the single assessment process for older people in England. *Primary Health Care Research and Development*, 11(1): 61–71.

Adams, T. 2008. *Dementia Care Nursing: Promoting Well-Being in People with Dementia and Their Families*. Basingstoke, UK: Palgrave MacMillan.

Alzheimer's Disease International. 2014. *World Alzheimer Report 2014: Dementia and Risk Reduction: An Analysis of Protective and Modifiable Factors*. London: Alzheimer's Disease International.

Boaden, R., Dusheiko, M., Gravelle, H., Parker, S., Pickard, S., Roland, M., Sargent, P., & Sheaff, R. 2006. *Evercare: Evaluations of the Evercare Approach to Case Management: Final Report*. Manchester, UK: National Primary Care Research and Development Centre.

Boult, C., Karm, L., & Groves, C. 2008. Improving chronic care: The 'Guided Care' model. *Permanente Journal*, 12(1): 50–54.

Cummings, N.A., Cummings, J.L., & Johnson, J.N. 1997. *Behavioral Health in Primary Care: A Guide for Clinical Integration*. Madison, CT: Psychosocial Press.

Curry, N., & Ham, C. 2010. *Clinical and Service Integration: The Route to Improved Outcomes*. London: King's Fund.

Department of Health. 2001. *National Service Framework for Older People*. London: Department of Health.

Department of Health. 2004. *The NHS Improvement Plan: Putting People at the Heart of Public Services*. London: Department of Health.

Department of Health. 2008. *Refocusing the Care Programme Approach: Policy and Positive Practice Guidance*. London: Department of Health.

Department of Health. 2009. *Living Well With Dementia: A National Dementia Strategy*. London: Department of Health.

Department of Health. 2010. *Equity and Excellence: Liberating the NHS*. London: Department of Health.

Department of Health. 2011. *No Health without Mental Health*. London: Department of Health.

Department of Health. 2012. *Prime Minister's Challenge on Dementia—Delivering Major Improvements in Dementia Care and Research by 2015*. London: Department of Health.

Department of Health. 2013. *Dementia—A State of the Nation Report on Dementia Care and Support in England*. London: Department of Health.

Department of Health. 2015. *Prime Minister's Challenge on Dementia 2020*. London: Department of Health.

Dutton, R. 2009. *Extra Care Housing and People with Dementia. What Do We Know About What Works Regarding the Built and Social Environment, and the Provision of Care and Support? A Scoping Review of the Literature 1998–2008: Version 1.7*. Worcester, UK: Housing and Dementia Research Consortium.

Ham, C., & Oldham, J. 2009. Integrating health and social care in England: Lessons from early adopters and implications for policy. *Journal of Integrated Care*, 17(6): 3–9.

Hutt, R., Rosen, R., & McCauley, J. 2004. *Case-Managing Long Term Conditions: What Impact Does It Have in the Treatment of Older People?* London: King's Fund.

International Value Cases. 2013. http://www.local.gov.uk/documents/10180/12193/ PACE+-+Driving+national+change+locally/e77a6eea-5e8d-46af-8d3d-a1d4499c2349.

Koch, T., Iliffe, S., Manthorpe, J., Stephens, B., Cox, C., Robinson, L., Livingston, G., et al. 2012. The potential of case management for people with dementia: A commentary. *International Journal of Geriatric Psychiatry*, 27(12): 1305–1313.

Lewis, G.H., Georghiou, T., Steventon, A., Vaithianathan, R., Chitnis, X., Billings, J., Blunt, I., et al. *Impact of 'Virtual Wards' on Hospital Use: A Research Study Using Propensity Matched Controls and a Cost Analysis*. London: National Institute for Health Research.

Mast, B. 2014. Whole person assessment and care planning. In *Excellence in Dementia Care*, 2nd edition, edited by Downs, M., & Bowers, B., 290–302. Maidenhead, UK: Open University Press.

Mental Capacity Act. 2005. http://www.legislation.gov.uk/ukpga/2005/9/contents.

Moniz-Cook, E., & Manthorpe, J. (Editors). 2009. *Early Psychological Interventions in Dementia: Evidence-Based Practice*. London: Kingsley.

National Collaborating Centre for Mental Health. 2007—Updated 2011. *Dementia: A NICE-SCIE Guideline on Supporting People with Dementia and Their Carers in Health and Social Care*. National Clinical Practice Guideline Number 42. Leicester, UK: British Psychological Society and Gaskell.

NHS England. 2014. *Commissioning for Quality and Innovation (CQUIN) 2014/15 Guidance*. London: NHS Commissioning Board.

Parker, D. 2012. Psychological interventions and working with the older adult. In *Psychological Interventions in Mental Health Nursing*, edited by Smith, G., 120–132. Maidenhead, UK: Open University Press.

Phillips, R.L., Han, M. Petterson, S.M., Makaroff, L., & Liaw, W.R. 2014. Cost, utilization, and quality of care: An evaluation of Illinois' Medicaid primary care case management program. *Annals of Family Medicine*, 12(5): 408–417.

Ross, S., Curry, N., & Goodwin, N. 2011. *Case Management. What Is It and How It Can Best Be Implemented*. London: King's Fund.

Wolff, J.L., Boyd, C.M., Reider, L., Palmer, S., Scharfstein, D., Marsteller, J., Wegener, S.T., et al. 2010. Effects of guided care on family caregivers. *The Gerontologist*, 50(4): 459–470.

Wolff, J.L., Giovannetti, E.R., Boyd, C.M., Reider, L., Palmer, S., Scharfstein, D., Marsteller, J., Wegener, S.T., Frey, K., Leff, B., & Frick, K.D. 2010. Effects of guided care on family caregivers. *The Gerontologist*, 50(4): 459–470.

Woods, L., Smith, G., Pendleton, J., & Parker, D. 2013. *Innovate Dementia Baseline Report*. Liverpool, UK: Liverpool John Moores University.

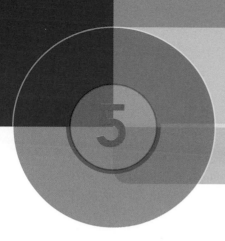

Risk management

REBECCA RYLANCE AND JAMES KIDD

AIMS

- To provide an overview of the types of risks that people living with dementia may encounter
- To explore a risk enablement framework utilising a strength-based approach via the use of a clinical scenario

OBJECTIVES

- To identify some of the pertinent risk factors for people who live with dementia and some of the relevant risk assessments
- Consideration of the safeguarding issues for people with dementia and their carers
- To examine a strength-based approach to maintain safety and maximise the well-being of people living with dementia

OVERVIEW

This chapter addresses risk, specifically the risks pertaining to people living with dementia. The word *risk* can mean different things to different people (Mitchell & Glendinning, 2007); arguably, professionals, carers and people living with dementia will interpret and understand 'risk' in different ways depending on their professional discipline (Department of Health [DH], 2010).

Broadly speaking, the concept of risk is the likelihood of an event occurring and how harmful it is likely to be should it occur (Morgan, 2000). Risk assessment is therefore the process of gathering and analysing information about a person to develop an understanding and evaluation of the person's unique risks (Rylance & Simpson, 2012). It follows, then, that risk management facilitates the opportunity for practitioners to intervene in a positive way that empowers people living with dementia and their carers to manage their own risks (DH, 2007).

However, managing risk is no easy task (Pratt, 2001); Clarke et al. (2009) argue that the management of risk in dementia care is far more complex than many other areas of clinical practice. It is often a challenge for carers and professionals to refrain from being overly protective and allowing a person living with dementia to have some power and control over their life (DH, 2010).

This chapter explores the types of risks that people who live with dementia may face and discusses the types of risk assessment and management approaches that are likely to be involved. The use of a clinical scenario helps underpin the principles of risk management from a strength-based perspective (as discussed later in the chapter).

TYPES OF RISKS

A typical mental health risk assessment should include consideration of the following domains (Harrison, 2003):

- Risk to self (suicide, self-harm, neglect)
- Risk of harm to others (dangerousness, forensic history)
- Risk from others to service user (abuse, harassment, exploitation)
- Risk of absconsion
- Risk of noncompliance with treatment
- Risk of substance misuse

Due to the complexity of dementia, vulnerability and most notably the high levels of co-morbidity that exist amongst people living with dementia, the risks are likely to be multifactorial and may differ to those presented by other mental health service users.

Examine the following scenario and identify the potential vulnerabilities or risks:

Sally is a 75-year-old woman who has recently returned home to her one-bedroom bungalow following a cerebrovascular accident (CVA) 3 months ago and a subsequent diagnosis of vascular dementia.

Her husband Jim reports that since her return home she appears to have difficulty concentrating and communicating. He also reports that Sally had been confused and occasionally aggressive. He claims that she 'keeps looking for the car keys to go out for a drive'. In response to this, he has hidden the car keys and put a bolt on the top of the front door to prevent her going out.

Unfortunately, Sally tried to unlock the bolt by climbing on a chair and fell off, sustaining minor injuries. This prompted Sally's husband to call her mental health practitioner.

Sally's husband is not in good health himself and is becoming worried.

Clearly, the risks in this scenario are complex and require thorough attention. The perceived risks may include:

- Is Sally at further risk of falling?
- Are speech and communication deteriorating?

- Are there risks of further cognitive decline?
- Are there dangers associated with driving a motor vehicle?
- Is there carer distress?
- Is there carer abuse?

In Sally's scenario she fell off her chair as a result of her husband Jim bolting the door. Before examining ways of managing this specific risk, the potential risks associated with her CVA should be explored. A physiotherapy and occupational therapist assessment would determine the potential risks around falls, mobility and any environmental hazards. It must be recognised that the risk of falling increases with age and cognitive impairment (Vassallo et al., 2009). Utilising simple risk assessment tools such as the STRATIFY Risk Assessment Tool (Oliver et al., 2004) and taking practical steps to improve the living environment can reduce and often prevent falls. Often, simple environmental changes such as night lights or removing trip hazards and obstacles can have a massive impact in terms of managing risk.

Impaired mobility could arise for a number of other reasons—for instance, as a physiological consequence of Sally's CVA or the side effects of some medications. Ensuring that medication is taken as prescribed and regular monitoring of any side effects should be an integral part of Sally's care. Having explored these potential risks, it is not apparent that Sally's mobility has been worsened by her CVA or treatment. Additional risks can emerge from the management of dementia. In Sally's scenario, her husband's attempt to 'keep her safe' by fixing a bolt high up on the door resulted in a new 'fall' risk.

Studies have shown that people living with dementia are more likely to experience dysphagia (Royal College of Speech & Language Therapists, 2005). In Sally's scenario, her husband reports that she appears to be having difficulty concentrating and communicating. Difficulties with social communication are a predominant feature in dementia and can reduce access to recreation, employment, or social integration, including forming relationships and expressing personality. This can have a major impact on the quality of life (Royal College of Speech & Language Therapists, 2013). A comprehensive speech and language therapy (SLT) assessment would ascertain whether Sally had any swallowing risks and what impact they may have on her ability to communicate.

Vascular dementia is a risk factor for impaired cognitive functioning. Approximately one-quarter of patients remain demented 3 months after a stroke (Haring, 2002). A large number of cognitive assessments are available, some better suited to community and some more suited to a hospital environment. Examples include the Abbreviated Mental Test Score (AMTS), 6 Item Cognitive Impairment Test (6CIT), General Practitioner Assessment of Cognition (GPCOG), Mini-Mental State Examination (MMSE), Addenbrooke's Cognitive Examination-111 (ACE-111), and Montreal Cognitive Assessment (MoCA). It is vital that Sally is regularly cognitively assessed by the team at her memory service, taking her husband's views into consideration.

The scenario states that Sally wishes to get into her car and drive, resulting in her husband hiding the keys. This can be a tricky situation; in fact, the Driver and Vehicle Licencing Agency (DVLA) published guidance on driving with dementia (DVLA, 2013). A diagnosis of dementia, however, is not necessarily a reason to stop driving—many people with dementia retain their driving skills and are able to drive safely for some years postdiagnosis. That said, certain legal requirements must be satisfied, including informing the DVLA and relevant insurance company. However, the issue concerns safety and whether a person living with dementia can continue to drive safely. It should be noted that a person with dementia will eventually lose his or her licence.

In Sally's case, her situation is compounded by her CVA and impaired mobility. Think for a moment about what you would do to keep Sally and other motorists safe. Did you know that Sally could be assessed at a regional mobility centre for a fee? Would you consider this option for Sally? If you did, what might the consequences be? Remember that if Sally is unsafe to drive, this may have a financial (in terms of taxis, public transport etc.) impact on her and her husband, as well as the consequences for Sally in terms of reduced independence. It may impact on Sally's husband further if he has to do more driving. This in turn could lead to significant carer distress.

Balancing the enormous task of caring for a person with dementia can demand skill, planning, patience and attention. By concentrating on Sally's needs alone, Jim may neglect his own health needs. As Sally's condition deteriorates and her needs change, it is likely that Jim will be less able to cope. The level of distress that carers experience, particularly in the later stages, should not be underestimated (Walker et al., 2007). Stressors for carers include:

- Denial (about the condition)
- Anger and frustration (Why is there no cure? Why does she keep repeating herself?)
- Guilt (Why do I lose my patience? She cannot help it.)
- Social isolation (It does feel it is not worth meeting friends and neighbours.)
- Anxiety (What does the future hold?)
- Depression and loss (loss of the former person, possibly loss of a sexual partner)
- Exhaustion (sleeping on the sofa, listening for Sally)
- Health problems (exacerbated angina)

Let us take a look at the scenario:

Sally's husband Jim has been sleeping on the sofa 'to keep an eye on the front door'. He reports that Sally gets up in the night and tries to leave the house. As a consequence of this, Jim is feeling extremely tired and confessed that he is 'not coping well'.

Jim also has angina and has been experiencing frequent chest pain, subsequently using his glyceryl trinitrate (GTN) spray more frequently.

A routine appointment with his GP resulted in Jim being referred to a cardiologist for a specialist check-up.

What might the consequences be for Sally if Jim goes to hospital? What are the consequences for Jim and his failing health? This scenario is not atypical—in fact the high morbidity that carers experience is well documented in the literature (National Institute for Health and Clinical Excellence [NICE], 2006; DH, 2009). A brief period of respite might be an option for them both. The National Dementia Strategy (DH, 2009: 12) points out the need for 'good quality personalised breaks' for carers (discussed later in this chapter).

It is therefore imperative that a comprehensive carer's assessment occur in tandem with assessment of Sally's needs. It is a fundamental right under the Carers (Equal Opportunities) Act (2004) that carers are given an assessment of needs. Furthermore, if a carer is experiencing psychological distress, he or she should be offered appropriate psychological therapy (NICE, 2006). It follows then that all care plans should have an intervention plan for the carer (as discussed later in the chapter).

Let us think for a moment about the possible support and interventions that can be offered to Jim. How about individual or group psycho-education? Training courses? Peer support and carer support groups? Telephone support (helplines)? Respite? Day/night sitting service? Can you think of any others? Even though health and social care managers should ensure that carers of people who live with dementia have access to a full range of supportive interventions, it is often difficult for the carer to 'let go'. Let us take a look at the scenario:

At Sally's last appointment at the Memory Clinic, the lead practitioner recommends that they attend the local hospital's postdiagnostic support group. They offer a 7-week course for people with dementia and their carers. The programme, which is cofacilitated by an occupational therapist and a psychologist, offers peer support and psycho-education on topics such as:

- Facts and myths about dementia
- Memory and how the brain works
- The impact of receiving a diagnosis
- Practical solutions to memory problems
- Wellness and well-being
- Future plans
- Resources for living well with dementia

Sally and Jim have also been assigned a 'care navigator' who can advise them both of relevant services and resources as needs and circumstances change.

A wealth of information and guidance about the risks of abuse associated with having a diagnosis of dementia is available (Cooper et al., 2009). However, much less is known about the abuse that people who informally care for people with dementia experience. Indeed it is probably massively under-reported, but it is an important factor to consider when assessing the risks for someone who is living with a progressive dementing condition.

Sally and Jim have been attending the postdiagnostic support group for 5 weeks and have made some new friends as well as receiving lots of support and information. They have subsequently joined a local walking group with some of the members, and Jim reports that Sally feels more tired in the evening and is sleeping much better.

On the occasions when Sally does wake up in the night, she often does not recognise Jim and appears to be quite frightened, repeatedly shouting at Jim to 'get away!' and sometimes lashing out with her hands.

A person living with dementia will often misidentify people (Mendez, 1992). This can often be hurtful and can be seen as a rejection by a carer, but keep in mind that the person living with dementia may not even recognise themselves.

When Sally does not recognise Jim, the risks of assault/abuse are greater. It is important that Jim seeks help and information to safeguard both his own and Sally's physical and psychological needs. Having looked at a variety of psychosocial risks for Sally and Jim, let us now move onto risk enablement.

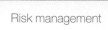
RISK ENABLEMENT: A STRENGTH-BASED APPROACH

Risk enablement is sometimes known as positive risk management. This is a process of identifying, assessing and addressing specific risk issues, while enablement is the principle underpinning the objective of that work. It involves weighing the potential benefits and harms of exercising one choice of action over another, identifying the potential risks involved, and developing plans and actions that reflect the positive potential and priorities of the service user (Morgan, 2004). Risk enablement is a strength-based approach that recognises each person living with dementia possesses more abilities than they have lost and builds on those abilities that he or she has retained. A strength-based approach to risk management does not mean ignoring challenges but instead focuses on a person's own strengths to create an environment where people are co-producers of support rather than passive consumers of support (Pattoni, 2012).

One of the biggest barriers to enabling people with dementia when managing risk is an overly cautious approach (DH, 2010). 'Safety first' approaches are disempowering for people with dementia (Clarke et al., 2009; Nuffield Council on Bioethics, 2009) and can prevent them from doing things that most people take for granted (DH, 2007). Blanket assumptions surrounding dementia are frequently made and this in turn can have a profound effect on how a person is perceived and treated by others, regardless of their actual capabilities. They may be excluded from discussions about their care because their views and preferences are not seen to be valid or are perceived to be a result of their condition (Manthorpe, 1997; Alzheimer's Society, 2013). Consequently, risk assessments often concentrate on minimising or eliminating risk without considering what aspect of independence, choice and potential might be lost (Nuffield Council on Bioethics, 2009). There is a risk, however, that in the process of management, people with dementia are put on the sidelines, seen as a hindrance, and have control taken away from them under the guise of it being 'for their own good'. Every effort should be made to listen, engage and work in partnership with the person living with dementia and his or her carer (DH, 2010; NICE, 2006).

Reflecting on the language used in positive risk management can be useful in orientating our perspective. 'Risk enablement', 'risk mitigation', and 'risk benefit assessments' are some suggestions for improving the way we talk about risk and can raise awareness of the balance that should be achieved in managing risk (DH, 2010). *Vulnerability* is a term that may be useful in indicating that a person may be at a higher level of risk from harm because of a disability or illness, but instead of thinking of them as *vulnerable people*, it might be better to think about how people with dementia often live in vulnerable *situations*. Let us revisit the scenario for a moment and consider what aspects of her daily routine that Sally can do for herself:

Jim tends to wake up first and takes Sally a cup of tea into the bedroom. He lays out her clothes for the day and prepares her toiletries in the bathroom. Other than a gentle reminder about the order that her clothes go on (i.e. cardigan over dress not vice versa), Sally manages to get herself dressed. Although Sally has had one or two episodes of incontinence (they have a supply of pads should they need them), Jim recognises when Sally goes looking for the bathroom and steers her towards it.

Can you identify a number of tasks that Sally can complete with minimal assistance? The scenario implies that with assistance Sally can get herself dressed and attend to her personal hygiene. It also suggests that Sally can have a cup of tea and take herself to the toilet. It is interesting that Jim recognises the subtle changes in Sally's behaviour when she is searching for the toilet. It is important that this type of information is communicated to health and social care professionals and clearly documented in care plans. Of paramount importance is that Sally continues to do as many things for herself for as long as possible (DH, 2009) and live well with dementia.

VULNERABILITY AND SAFEGUARDING

Although Sally's scenario does not overtly imply that any abuse is occurring, it is still important to recognise that people with dementia are especially vulnerable because the disease may prevent them from recognising abuse or reporting abuse. In a UK study, a third of family carers of people with dementia reported abusive behaviour towards the person for whom they are caring (Cooper et al., 2009). Two international studies found overall rates of abuse of people with dementia by their caregivers ranging from 34% to 62% (Cooney, Howard, & Lawlor, 2006; Yan & Kwok, 2011). While there is a large body of literature which addresses safeguarding an *adult at risk* in organisational and professional settings, there is less guidance available where the person is living in the family home and support is provided by family members.

Safeguarding in a family setting can be considered from two perspectives: abuse that is perpetrated deliberately and abuse that is not. Sometimes the family member is doing his or her best but cannot provide the level of care and support that is needed or hasn't the knowledge to apply the principles which underpin enablement. Regardless of whether or not the abuse is perpetrated deliberately, from the perspective of the victim the impact is the same. For this reason, all forms of abuse are unacceptable and equally subject to the law (Alzheimer's Society, 2013).

Let us take a step back for a moment and revisit an extract from Sally's scenario:

He [Jim] claims that she 'keeps looking for the car keys to go out for a drive'. In response to this, he has hidden the car keys and put a bolt on the top of the front door to prevent her going out.

Unfortunately, Sally tried to unlock the bolt by climbing on a chair and fell off, sustaining minor injuries.

Is it OK to lock the front door of the house to prevent Sally from going outside at night?

Although Sally is sleeping much better since joining the walking group, Jim still sleeps on the sofa for 'peace of mind', and having put a bolt on Sally's bedroom door, he is getting a good night's sleep himself.

In both scenarios, Jim has used a locked door to curtail Sally's movements around the bungalow. Would locking a front door be considered abusive? Do you lock your front door at night? It is unlikely that locking a front door at night would be classed as abusive. However, would locking a person in their room at night be a form of abuse? The answer is that it could be. While some aspects of abuse are often clear cut, such as financial abuse, other aspects, such as depriving a person of freedom of movement, are not. Abuse which is not deliberate can include a wide range of actions, including neglect or the unnecessary confinement of a person with dementia. The general principle in restricting people's freedom of movement is the *least restrictive* option (Mental Capacity Act, 2005).

Working with families and loved ones who provide care must be a collaborative enterprise (NICE, 2006). It is important not to dismiss carers' concerns or solutions to the problems that they identify. In this case we might keep the option of locking Sally's bedroom at night as a possible solution, but work backwards and try to identify what risks Jim's management solution is intended to address. There could be a number of reasons why Sally wants to go out or move around the bungalow. Once you identify what Sally is trying to achieve, you can start to generate a range of options and ways to meet her needs. When working with service users and their families it is essential to take a holistic view.

MAINTAINING SAFETY AND MAXIMIZING WELL-BEING

It is possible to live well with dementia. The National Dementia Strategy in '*Living Well with Dementia*' (DH, 2009) claims that all people living with dementia and those who care for them will have the best possible health care and support. The strategy set out a national framework outlining the proposed transformation of dementia services including such things as timely access to diagnosis, education and information for patients and carers and easy access to good quality health and social care. This ultimately calls for massive societal change. Since the publication of this document there have been many national campaigns to help implement and embed the strategy.

In terms of Sally and Jim, we have previously discussed that they have joined a walking club, which will undoubtedly have health benefits both physically and psychologically (Erickson et al., 2011; Scarmeas et al., 2009). Let us look at how they are getting on:

Sally and Jim completed the postdiagnostic support group at their local hospital, where they made some new friends. They are both well informed about Sally's condition and have since told other family members and friends, who have been supportive.

Sally decided not to drive anymore but can still manage to get around on the bus and the local taxi service if she has to but tends to rely on Jim.

A couple who are old friends now come over every second Tuesday of each month. The woman takes Sally to the local garden centre for a look around and some lunch, and Jim and the man go for a nine-hole game of golf.

Jim and Sally still walk weekly with their walking group, and Sally has been discharged by the stroke team on account of her improved mobility. They have also joined a social group called 'Enjoy the Memories', which is hosted at a local football club and offers reminiscence workshops, cookery courses, custom-made life story books and day trips to local places of interest.

The social environment is so important for Sally and Jim. The richness of interactions and relationships can significantly improve quality of life for people who live with dementia (DH, 2009). Humans have a basic fundamental need for social connectedness (Cacioppo & Patrick,

2009), and a person living with dementia should not have to live with reduced social vitality. Sally is living well with dementia and Jim is feeling less stressed and better able to cope. Most people want to live in their own home for as long as possible, and most family carers want to continue to support their loved one to stay at home, but they often need assistance and respite (DH, 2009).

By working collaboratively with both Sally and Jim (coordinated by health and social care agencies) and by ensuring that care plans are person centred/relationship centred, Sally will live at home for as long as possible. By focussing on what she can do rather than what she cannot do and having risk assessment and management plans that focus on that, Sally and Jim can continue to live well together for some time.

CHAPTER SUMMARY

This chapter examined the types of risks that people who live with dementia may encounter in their day-to-day life.

We looked at a number of specific risk assessment tools, and via the use of a clinical scenario we explored and discussed the risks for a person living with dementia at home.

We considered the safeguarding and vulnerability issues for both people who live with dementia and their carers, and by utilising a risk enablement framework and developing a strength-based approach throughout the scenario, we identified a number of strategies to maximise well-being and help a person live well with dementia.

REFLECTION ON LEARNING

1. Risk assessment is the process of gathering and analysing information about a person to evaluate their unique risk. True or false?
2. People with vascular dementia have fewer risks generally. True or false?
3. It is not possible to drive when a person has a diagnosis of dementia. True or false?
4. Informal carers of people with dementia can often experience significant psychological distress. True or false?
5. It is important to assist people with dementia to do as much as possible for themselves. True or false?
6. People with dementia are at risk of abuse. True or false?
7. Carers of people with dementia are at risk of abuse. True or false?
8. Diet and exercise are unimportant for people who live with dementia. True or false?
9. People with dementia are unable to maintain social relationships. True or false?
10. It is possible to live well with dementia. True or false?

REFERENCES

Alzheimer's Society. 2013. *The Dementia Guide. Living Well after Diagnosis.* London: Alzheimer's Society.

Carers (Equal Opportunities) Act. 2004. Chapter 15. London: HMSO. Available at http://www. legislation.gov.uk/ukpga/2004/15/contents

Cacioppo, J.T., & Patrick, W. 2009. *Loneliness: Human Nature and the Need for Social Connection.* London: Norton.

Clarke, C.L., Gibb, C.E., Keady, J., Luce, A., Wilkinson, H., Williams, L., & Cook, A. 2009. Risk management dilemmas in dementia care: An organizational survey in three UK countries. *International Journal of Older People Nursing*, 4: 89–96.

Cooney, C., Howard, R., & Lawlor, B. 2006. Abuse of vulnerable people with dementia by their carers: Can we identify those most at risk? *International Journal of Geriatric Psychiatry*, 21: 564–571.

Cooper, C., Selwood, A., Blanchard, M., Walker, Z., Blizard, R., & Livingston, G. 2009. Abuse of people with dementia by family carers: Representative cross-sectional study. *British Medical Journal*, 338. doi:http://dx.doi.org/10.1136/bmj.b155.

Department of Health. 2005. Mental Capacity Act. London: HMSO. Available at www.legislation.gov.uk/ukpga/2005/9/contents

Department of Health. 2007. *Best Practice in Managing Risk: Principles and Evidence for Best Practice in the Assessment and Management of Risk to Self and Others in Mental Health Services.* London: HMSO.

Department of Health. 2009. *Living Well with Dementia: A National Dementia Strategy.* London: HMSO.

Department of Health. 2010. *Nothing ventured nothing gained.* London: HMSO.

Driver and Vehicle Licencing Agency. 2013. *DVLA's Current Medical Guidelines For Professionals—Conditions A–C.* London: HMSO.

Erickson, K.l., Voss, M.W., Prakash, R.S., Basak, C., Szabo, A., Chaddock, L., Kim, J.S., et al. 2011. Exercise training increases size of hippocampus and improves memory. *Proceedings of the National Academy of Sciences of the United States of America*, 108(7): 3017–3022.

Haring, H.P. 2002. Cognitive impairment after stroke. *Current Opinion in Neurology*, 15: 79–84.

Harrison, A. 2003. A guide to risk assessment. *Nursing Times*, 99(9): 44–45.

Manthorpe, J. 1997. Elderly abuse and key areas in social work. In *The Mistreatment of Elderly People*, 2nd edition, edited by Decalmer, P., & Glendinning, F., 88–101. London: Sage.

Mendez, M.F. 1992. Delusional misidentification of persons in dementia. *British Journal of Psychiatry*, 160(3): 414–416.

Mitchell, W., & Glendinning, C. 2007. *A Review of the Research Evidence Surrounding Risk Perceptions, Risk Management Strategies and Their Consequences in Adult Social Care for Different Groups of Service Users.* York, UK: University of York, Social Policy Research Unit.

Morgan, S. 2000. *Clinical Risk Management: A Clinical Tool and Practitioner Manual.* London: Sainsbury Centre for Mental Health.

Morgan, S. 2004. Strength-based practice. *Open Mind*, 126: 16–17.

National Institute for Health and Clinical Excellence. 2006. *Dementia. Supporting People with Dementia and Their Carers in Health and Social Care.* Nice Clinical Guideline 42. London: NICE.

Nuffield Council on Bioethics. 2009. *Dementia: Ethical Issues.* London: Nuffield Council on Bioethics.

Oliver, D., Daly, F., Martin, F.C., & McCurdo, M.E.T. 2004. Risk factors and risk assessment tools for falls in hospital inpatients: A systematic review. *Age & Aging*, 33(2): 122–130.

Pattoni, L. 2012. *Insights 16: Strength-Based Approaches for Working with Individuals.* Glasgow: Institute for Research and Innovation in Social Services.

Pratt, D. 2001. Risk management in mental health. *Nursing Times*, 97(25): 37–38.

Royal College of Speech and Language Therapists. 2005. *Speech and Language Therapy Provision for People with Dementia: Position Paper.* London: RCSLT.

Royal College of Speech and Language Therapists. 2013. *Resource Manual for Commissioning and Planning Services for Speech, Language and Communication Needs.* London: RCSLT.

Rylance, R., & Simpson, P. 2012. Psychological interventions and managing risk. In *Psychological Interventions in Mental Health Nursing,* edited by Smith, G., 11–23. Maidenhead, UK: Open University Press.

Scarmeas, N., Luchsinger, J.A., Schupt, N., Brickman, A.M., Cosentino, S., Tang, M.X., & Stern, Y. 2009. Physical activity, diet and risk of Alzheimer's disease. *Journal of the American Medical Association,* 302(6): 627–637.

Vassallo, M., Mallela, S.K., Williams, A., Kwan, J., Allens, S., & Sharma, J.C. 2009. Fall risk factors in elderly patients with cognitive impairment on rehabilitation wards. *Geriatrics & Gerontology International,* 9(1): 41–46.

Walker, A.E., Livingston, G., Cooper, C.A., Katona, C.L.E., & Kitchen, G.L. 2007. Caregivers' experience of risk in dementia: The LASER-AD Study. *Ageing & Mental Health,* 10(5): 532–538.

Yan, E., & Kwok, T. 2011. Abuse of older Chinese with dementia by family caregivers: An inquiry into the role of caregiver burden. *International Journal of Geriatric Psychiatry,* 26(5): 527–535.

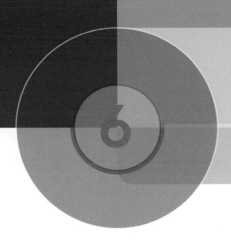

Living well with dementia

GRAHAME SMITH, JACKIE DAVENPORT, AND
DENISE PARKER

AIM

- To explore in depth the notion of living well with dementia

OBJECTIVES

- To consider living well with dementia as a pathway towards a person being and feeling independent
- To identify and evaluate the component parts of living well with dementia, which include meaningful activity, the environment, nutrition, and daylight

OVERVIEW

Based on current estimates, two-thirds of the 835,000 people with dementia in the UK live in the community; the majority live in their own homes, with some living alone (Alzheimer's Society, 2014). Living with dementia not only has a profound impact on the person with dementia but also has a profound impact on informal carers, who are normally family members (Woods et al., 2013; Alzheimer's Society, 2014). The prime carer is frequently an older adult who may be physically frail. They often experience high levels of stress. The challenges they deal with can lead to a decreased quality of life (Department of Health [DH], 2009; Woods et al., 2013). It is important to recognise that

> … caring cuts across the age range and in some cases might be undertaken by children or young people under 18. (DH, 2009: 17)

Living well with dementia is an admirable aspiration for society as a whole. To enable this aspiration to be a reality it must be acknowledged that

… people with dementia and family carers can live well if they have access to good quality, integrated care that is affordable, and if they live in a housing environment that meets their needs. (Alzheimer's Society, 2014: "Executive Summary")

A starting place for this societal aspiration to become a reality has been the development of a number of national dementia strategies both within the UK and within the European Union. As an example, the DH's (2009) National Dementia Strategy aims to

… ensure that significant improvements are made to dementia services across three key areas: improved awareness, earlier diagnosis and intervention, and a higher quality of care. The Strategy identifies 17 key objectives which, when implemented, largely at a local level, should result in significant improvements in the quality of services provided to people with dementia and should promote a greater understanding of the causes and consequences of dementia. (DH, 2009: "Executive Summary")

Building on this strategy, there have been a number of initiatives across the UK to promote the message of living well with dementia. The Dementia Friends campaign is one of these initiatives which aims to recruit a million Dementia Friends by 2015. Dementia Friends will not only have a better understanding of dementia but also will be urged to turn understanding into action (Woods et al., 2013). To explore living well with dementia at a more practical level, this chapter examines and develops the following scenario:

John is a student nurse caring for Mrs Swift, who has dementia. She lives at home and is normally cared for by her husband. John is currently studying a dementia module for his nursing degree and is keen to ensure that any negative impact of Mrs Swift's hospital admission is minimised.

ENABLING INDEPENDENCE

Enable people with dementia and their carers to live well with dementia by the provision of good-quality care for all with dementia from diagnosis to the end of life, in the community, in hospitals and in care homes. (DH, 2009: 21)

A number of developments related to the enabling of independent living focus on people living with dementia being centrally involved. This includes projects such as the EDUCATE (Early Dementia Users' Co-operative Aiming to Educate) project (Woods et al., 2013). As part of this project people with dementia share their experiences in the role of educator at training events and aim to positively influence policies and promote improved services (North West Joint Improvement Partnership, 2010; Woods et al., 2013). Another example is DEEP (Dementia Engagement and Empowerment Programme). This project empowers and engages people living with dementia by collating views on how services and culture can be changed to meet real needs (Williamson, 2012; Woods et al., 2013).

Listening to people with dementia is a key part of understanding their meaning of living well and also their meaning of what it is to be independent (Kitwood, 1997). The DH (2009) takes the view that independent living relates to a nonreliance on 'more intensive services'. This form of independent living includes supporting the use of different housing options and the use of assistive technology (DH, 2009).

Housing options range from supportive services which enable people with dementia to stay at home and are layered on conventional housing to purpose-built accommodation where support services are integrated within the design of the building (Regnier & Denton, 2009; Woods et al., 2013). Assistive technologies can support independence by contributing to a person's sense of security, such as the ability to call for help in an emergency (Woods et al., 2013; Alladice, 2005). In most cases assistive technologies are used within the home setting as an additional service. In purpose-built accommodation, assistive technology is part of the design of the building (Woods et al., 2013; Gibson et al., 2014).

Delivering support services within the home setting which enable a person to be independent needs to be based on a flexible approach—one that is 'fit for the future' (Woods et al., 2013). Services will have to be adaptive to people living in different types of housing. This includes maintaining a person's independence while an inpatient in preparation for the person returning home, having different types of assistive technology available throughout a person's care journey, and ensuring good quality care is affordable and sustainable (Ham, Dixon, & Brooke, 2012). Let us return to John:

John wants to ensure Mrs Swift's independence is not compromised while she is an inpatient. He makes sure Mr and Mrs Swift are both involved in planning her care, and documents this carefully. Mr Swift gives John his wife's 'This Is Me' document from a previous admission (Alzheimer's Society, 2013). This provides a 'snapshot' of the person with dementia, giving information about the person as an individual such as preferences, likes, dislikes and interests. John updates this with the couple and obtains permission to share it with other staff. He then orientates them to the ward, showing them the toilet and the nurses' station.

MEANINGFUL ACTIVITY

The evidence consistently suggests that people with dementia experience poorer health and wellbeing outcomes than their counterparts without the condition. (Alzheimer's Society, 2014: 29)

On the basis of the above it is important that people with dementia are supported to have and maintain a healthy lifestyle (Young & Illsley, 2014; Woods et al., 2013; National Collaborating Centre for Mental Health, 2007/2011). This includes empowering people living with dementia to make informed choices and decisions about activities and interventions that are available (DH, 2011; Woods et al., 2013). Young and Illsley (2014) made the point that there are a number of evidence-based interventions available that promote health and help to prevent disease; these include:

- Diet
- Prevention of heart attacks and stroke

- Promoting activity
- Flu prevention
(Young & Illsley, 2014: 257)

This health promotion message should start before the onset of the condition. There is little evidence for its role in the prevention of dementia, though it has to be acknowledged that physical exercise still has a positive impact on people with dementia by improving their quality of life and their physical health, and in some cases slowing the progression of their symptoms (Woods et al., 2013; Foster, Rosenblatt, & Kuljis, 2011; Young & Illsley, 2014). Irrespective of age or whether a person has a dementia diagnosis, being active—especially physically active—has health benefits (Young & Illsley, 2014; World Health Organisation, 2010). Physical activity covers a range of exercises including walking, yoga, tai chi, cycling, stretching and toning, chair-based and multimodal exercises. Aerobic exercise is currently viewed as more beneficial than stretching and toning exercises (Woods et al., 2013; Forbes et al., 2008; Colombe & Kramer, 2003; Lautenschlager, 2008; Erickson et al., 2011).

There is a large variation in recommendations for the content, intensity, frequency and length of an exercise programme (Scarmeas et al., 2011; Fang et al., 2013; Abbot et al., 2004; Erickson, 2010; Lautenschlager, 2008). Currently it is recommended an older adult (over 65) should engage in 30 minutes of exercise at least five times per week and engage in a physical activity which improves muscle strength on at least two days a week (Department of Health, Physical Activity, Health Improvement and Protection, 2011). Activity is not only about physical exercise—engaging in social activities that include intellectual, cognitive and social stimulation are just as important, though there has to be a balance between under- and overstimulation (Foster, Rosenblatt, & Kuljis, 2011; Woods et al., 2013; Perrin & May, 2000; Verbeek et al., 2008).

Mr Swift is pleased that Mrs Swift appears to have settled well on the ward as he says she gets upset easily. During the afternoon Mrs Swift twice mistakes the linen room door for the toilet door and becomes distressed when it is locked. John does not want Mrs Swift to stop being active, as he is aware of the health benefits. He starts to think about how this problem could be overcome:

- There could be a larger, brighter sign on the toilet door.
- There could be brighter lighting in the corridor.
- There could be a pathway of LED lights in the floor from each bay to the toilet door.

John puts his ideas to the charge nurse.

THE ENVIRONMENT

Ideally a person with dementia would 'age in place'. In other words the person would continue to live in his or her home setting until the end of life. Due to the way services are provided this is not always easy to achieve (Woods et al., 2013; Lawton, 1997). Irrespective of the care setting, to be therapeutic the environment should be comforting, safe and understandable (Woods et al., 2013; Zeisel et al., 2003; Dijkstra, Pieterse, & Pruyn, 2006). A well-designed environment can enable a person with dementia to have a good quality of life by reducing agitation and dependence, while at the same time promoting social contact. To achieve this the designer needs to listen and understand what it is like to live with dementia (Chaudhury & Cooke, 2014; Lawton, 2001).

There are a number of models which conceptualise the relationship between a person with dementia and their environment. Chaudhury and Cooke (2014) describe the following as the three main theories:

- Individual competence and environmental press
- Model of place
- Progressively lower threshold

All three theories are helpful in understanding that a person with dementia interacts dynamically with their environment. Taking this into account the health and social care practitioner has to consider a person's competence, how the person's condition is having an impact on his or her ability to function, whether the environment is too challenging and difficult to negotiate, how the person is experiencing the environment, or if the environment is stressful for the individual. By taking these factors into consideration the practitioner can provide an environment that enables a person with dementia to have a good quality of life and contributes to avoiding increased disability (Woods et al., 2013; Chaudhury & Cooke, 2014). It is not always possible to sufficiently adapt a person's current home in order that a move to residential care can be prevented. Where this type of care is required there should be a concerted effort to ensure the physical environment is person centred (Woods et al., 2013; Chaudhury & Cooke, 2014). Chenoweth et al. (2014) highlight that a person-centred environment has safe, accessible outdoor and indoor spaces which enhance social interaction through the use of colour and provides 'objects for way-finding and to improve feelings of familiarity' (p. 1150).

Now, let us return to the example of John:

The charge nurse is delighted with John's ideas for trying to enable independence for the increasing numbers of people with dementia coming into the care of the National Health Service (NHS). The charge nurse thinks that lack of money will be the main obstacle but suggests that John contact the estates manager to discuss his ideas.

The estates manager indicates the following:

- Bright signs which are consistent throughout the ward can be ordered for the toilet doors at minimal cost.
- Although cost prohibits new lighting in the corridor, the estates manager will put brighter bulbs in the light fixtures outside the toilets.
- Infrastructure and cost prohibit an LED pathway (though John's idea has impressed all the staff). However, the estates manager knows that in accident and emergency (A&E) pathways of different coloured adhesive spots on the floor are used to guide patients to x-ray, fracture clinic or minor injury clinics, and these have been successful. He thinks that coloured spots from the bays to the toilets will not be a problem and can be implemented quickly.

NUTRITION

> Individuals with dementia frequently lose weight whether they are cared for at home, in hospital or in a long-term care facility. (Cole, 2012: 47)

Dementia can impact in different ways on a person's nutritional experience. Generally people with dementia may experience weight loss or weight gain, undernutrition, and dehydration (Woods et al., 2013; DH, 2009). Similar to exercise, nutritional advice as a health promotion and prevention message is becoming more prevalent within the dementia field (DH, 2009; Woods et al., 2013). Young and Illsley (2014) highlight that eating a healthy diet which includes eating at least five portions of fruit and vegetables a day is just as relevant to people with dementia, especially where there is a risk of stroke or coronary heart disease.

To understand a person's nutritional needs it is essential that there is a robust assessment process which acknowledges the importance of a person's identity, cultural needs, and likes and dislikes, and identifies any eating difficulties (Woods et al., 2013; DH, 2001). The challenge for the health and social care practitioner is that though there are a number of assessment tools in use within the dementia field, there is not one that fits all needs (Woods et al., 2013; Green & Watson, 2006). There is a pressing need for further research in this area and there are a number of promising studies which will help in the process of determining the correct nutritional elements and levels for people with dementia (Lim et al., 2006; Sydenham et al., 2012; Malouf, Grimley, & Areosa, 2008; De Jager et al., 2012; Llwellyn et al., 2009; Scheltens et al., 2012). In the meantime the health and social care practitioner should consider the following (Cole, 2012):

- Extra staff time and training have a positive effect on nutritional intake.
- The presence of registered nurses during mealtimes is important not only to assist in the feeding of people who have established eating difficulties but also to observe those who are developing eating difficulties.
- Engaging the advice of a dietician, introduction of nutritional supplements, allowing extra time for the person to eat his or her meal and providing assistance with feeding before dietary intake declines dramatically are also important factors. (Cole, 2012: 48)

As a person's dementia progresses they can experience difficulties in swallowing. According to Parker and Power (2013), these difficulties can initially arise in part from a person 'forgetting when they last ate, having trouble recognising food, eating too quickly or too slowly, and not being able to articulate their food preferences' (p. 26). As the condition becomes advanced, swallowing difficulties relate more to physiological changes (Parker & Power, 2013) such as 'delays in the swallow trigger, reduced movement of the larynx to protect the airway, and generalised pharyngeal weakness' (p. 26).

Returning to John:

John encourages Mrs Swift to have a walk around the ward before her meals. Being able to find the toilet means she can wash her hands before meals, something that is indicated in her 'This Is Me' document as part of her usual routine. Because she can do this, she is also less distressed, and this makes helping her to eat her meals much easier for her and the staff.

DAYLIGHT

Even though light as a therapy is not recommended, the NICE [National Institute for Health and Clinical Excellence] (2011) guidelines for dementia suggest using high light levels and providing access to natural light. This is with a focus on improving an individual's sleep-wake cycle. (Smith, 2014: 14)

There is promising evidence that light has a crucial role to play in the management of distressing symptoms such as agitation and aggression and disordered sleep (Woods et al., 2013; Vardy, & Robinson, 2011; Azermai et al., 2012; Smith, 2014). Using light as an intervention in dementia is in its early stages. However, due to its increasing use it is important that the health and social care practitioner understand its value within their practice (Woods et al., 2013; Smith, 2014). The move away from being reliant on pharmacological interventions in the field of dementia has led to a greater consideration of such approaches as light therapy (Smith, 2014):

The interest in using light as an intervention or light as therapy has arisen from noticing that distressing symptoms in dementia such as agitation and aggression can be worse at certain times of the day, commonly the late afternoon to evening—also known as the 'sundowning phenomena'. (Smith, 2014: 12)

At a neurological level light therapy works in part by inhibiting melatonin and therefore reducing drowsiness (Smith, 2014). Light therapy is not meant to be a substitute for daylight. If people with dementia can access daylight all the better; where this is difficult, then lighting which is equivalent to daylight should be considered (Smith, 2014). Similar to daylight, this type of light should be consistent with a normalised rest-wake cycle with lighting levels peak during the day and then start to recede as day progresses to night (Smith, 2014; Carvalho-Bos et al., 2007). Using light in this way can assist in the effective management of a person's sleep pattern. It also can potentially lead to a reduction in agitated-type behaviour by reducing drowsiness and improving cognition (Woods et al., 2013; Smith, 2014).

Similarly, improving light quality enables people with dementia to make better sense of their environment. This can help in reducing a person's frustration and will also assist in the prevention of falls (Voermans et al., 2007, 2013; Hughes & Adams, 2012). Using light to manage sleep, agitation and aggression, and in the prevention of falls is an approach that works well within a hospital or a residential environment, especially where a practitioner is trained to use this type of intervention (Smith, 2014). The challenge lies in using light as an intervention within the home environment, especially where a person with dementia does not have sufficient access to daylight or good-quality lighting conditions (Woods et al., 2013; Smith, 2014; Cook, 2012; Carswell et al., 2009; McCullagh et al., 2009; McGilton et al., 2007).

John is pleased he spoke up about his ideas. Toilets are more clearly indicated on the ward following the interventions, and the lighting conditions on the ward have been improved. The estates manager was enthused about improving the environment to support enabling independence for people with dementia and has also had the architrave around all the toilet doors painted a bright white.

CHAPTER SUMMARY

There have been a number of initiatives across the UK to promote the message of living well with dementia. At a strategic level, independent living relates to nonreliance on more intensive services which include residential services at a personal level. It relates to listening to people with dementia to understand their opinion of what it is to be independent.

The evidence shows that preventing and managing dementia is multifaceted, with strategies still emerging or to be confirmed. For these strategies to be successful and enable people with dementia to be independent they need to be based on a flexible approach that is fit for the future.

It is important that people with dementia are supported to have and maintain a healthy lifestyle. The role of the health and social practitioner is to empower people living with dementia to make informed choices and decisions about activities and interventions that are available. This approach has to be personalised, especially when considering a person's nutritional needs, as dementia can impact in different ways on a person's nutritional experience.

Preferably, a person with dementia would age in place and be supported to live in their home setting until the end of life; irrespective of the care setting, the environment has to be comforting, safe and understandable. There is promising evidence that light as an environmental intervention has a crucial role to play in the management of distressing symptoms in dementia. The use of light in this way is in its early stages; however, due to its increasing use, it is important that the health and social care practitioner recognise its value within their practice.

REFLECTION ON LEARNING

1. Statistically, where do people with dementia live?
2. What is the aim of the Dementia Friends initiative?
3. Strategically, how is independent living defined?
4. Why is listening important, and what does it help the health and social care practitioner understand?
5. List the evidence-based interventions that promote healthy lifestyles.
6. Currently, which exercise is viewed as more beneficial for people with dementia?
7. List the three main theories which conceptualise the relationship between a person with dementia and the person's environment.
8. To understand the nutritional needs of a person with dementia, what must the health and social care practitioner do?
9. List the psychological and physiological changes a person with dementia experiences that can impact negatively on their ability to swallow.
10. Which is better, daylight or artificial light?

REFERENCES

Abbot, R.D., White, L.R., Ross, G.W., Masaki, K.H., Curb, J.D., & Petrovich, H. 2004. Walking and dementia in physically capable elderly men. *JAMA*, 292: 1447–1453.

Alladice, J. 2005. A 20/20 Vision for Housing and Care. http://www.cih.org/policy/2020Report.pdf.

Alzheimer's Society. 2013. This Is Me Tool. http://www.alzheimers.org.uk/site/scripts/download_info.php?fileID=1604.

Alzheimer's Society. 2014. *Dementia 2014: Opportunity for Change*. London: Alzheimer's Society.

Azermai, M., Petrovica, M., Elseviers, M.M., Bourgeois, J., Van Bortel, L.M., & Vander Stichele, R.H. 2012. Systematic appraisal of dementia guidelines for the management of behavioural and psychological symptoms. *Ageing Research Reviews*, 11: 78–86.

Carswell, W., McCullagh, P.J., Augusto, J.C., Martin, S., Mulvenna, M.D., Zheng, H., Wang, H.Y., et al. 2009. A review of the role of assistive technology for people with dementia in the hours of darkness. *Technology and Health Care*, 17: 1–24.

Carvalho-Bos, S.S., Riemersma-van der Lek, R.F., Waterhouse, J., Reilly, T., & Van Someren, E.J.W. 2007. Strong association of the rest–activity rhythm with well-being in demented elderly women. *American Journal of Geriatric Psychiatry*, 15: 92–100.

Chaudhury, H., & Cooke, H. 2014. Design matters in dementia care: The role of the physical environment in dementia care settings. In *Excellence in Dementia Care*, 2nd edition, edited by Downs, M., & Bowers, B., 144–158. Maidenhead, UK: Open University Press.

Chenoweth, L., Forbes, I., Fleming, R., King, M.T., Stein-Parbury, J., Luscombe, G., Kenny, P., Jeon, Y.-H., Haas, M., & Brodaty, H. 2014. PerCEN: A cluster randomized controlled trial of person-centered residential care and environment for people with dementia. *International Psychogeriatrics*, 26(7): 1147–1160.

Cole, D. 2012. Optimising nutrition for older people with dementia. *Nursing Standard*, 26(20): 41–48.

Colombe, S., & Kramer, A F. 2003. Fitness effects on the cognitive function of older adults; a meta-analytic study. *Psychological Science*, 14(2): 125–130.

Cook, D.J. 2012. How smart is your home? *Science*, 335(30): 1579–1581.

de Jager, C., Oulhaj, A , Jacoby, R., Refsum, H., & Smith, A.D. 2012. Cognitive and clinical outcomes of homocysteine-lowering B-vitamin treatment in mild cognitive impairment: A randomized controlled trial. *International Journal of Geriatric Psychiatry*, 27: 592–600.

Department of Health. 2001. *Treatment Choice in Psychological Therapies and Counselling. Evidence Based Clinical Practice Guideline*. London: Department of Health.

Department of Health. 2009. *Living Well with Dementia: A National Dementia Strategy*. London: Department of Health.

Department of Health. (2011). *NHS Operating Framework 2012–13*. London: Department of Health.

Department of Health, Physical Activity, Health Improvement and Protection. 2011. *Start Active, Stay Active: A Report on Physical Activity from the Four Home Countries' Chief Medical Officers*. London: Department of Health.

Dijkstra, K., Pieterse, M., & Pruyn, A. 2006. Physical environmental stimuli that turn healthcare facilities into healing environments through psychologically mediated effects: Systematic review. *Journal of Advanced Nursing*, 56(2): 166–181.

Erickson, K.I., Voss, M.W., Prakash, R.S., Basak, C., Szabo, A., & Chaddock. 2011. Exercise training increases size of hippocampus and improves memory. *Proceedings of the National Academy of Sciences of the United States of America*, 108(7): 3017–3022.

Fang, Y., Nelson, N.W., Savik, K., Wyman, J.F., Dysken, M. & Bronas, U.G. 2013. Affecting cognition and quality of life via aerobic exercise in Alzheimer's disease. *Western Journal of Nursing Research*, 35(1): 24–38.

Forbes, D., Forbes, S., Morgan, D.G., Markle-Reid, M., Wood, J., & Culum, I. 2008. Physical activity programs for persons with dementia. *Cochrane Database of Systematic Reviews*, (3). doi:10.1002/14651858.CD006489.pub2.

Foster, P.P., Rosenblatt, K.P., & Kuljis, R.O. 2011. Exercise–induced cognitive plasticity, implications for mild cognitive impairment and Alzheimer's disease. *Frontiers in Neurology*, 2(28). doi:10.3389/fneur.2011.00028.

Gibson, G., Newton, L., Pritchard, G., Finch, T., Brittain, K., & Robinson, L. 2014. The provision of assistive technology products and services for people with dementia in the United Kingdom. *Dementia*, 0(0): 1–21: doi:10.1177/1471301214532643.

Green, S.M., & Watson, R.N. 2006. Nutritional screening and assessment tools for older adults: A literature review. *Journal of Advanced Nursing*, 54(4): 477–490.

Ham, C., Dixon, A., & Brooke, B. 2012. *Transforming the Delivery of Health and Social Care*. London: Kings Fund.

Hughes, L., & Adams, L. 2012. Non-pharmaceutical approach to managing behavioural disturbances in patients with dementia in a nursing home setting. *BMC Proceedings*, 6(4): 7.

Kitwood, T. 1997. *Dementia Reconsidered*. London: Open University Press.

Lautenschlager, N.T. 2008. Physical activity improves cognitive function in people with memory impairments. *Journal of the American Medical Association*, 300: 1027–1037.

Lawton, M.P. 1997. Assessing quality of life in Alzheimer disease research. *Alzheimer Disease and Associated Disorders*, 11(6): 91–99.

Lawton, M.P. 2001. The physical environment of the person with Alzheimer's disease. *Aging & Mental Health*, 5(Supplement 1): 56–64.

Lim, W.S., Gammack, J.K., Van Niekerk, K., & Dangour, A. 2006. Omega 3 fatty acid for the prevention of dementia. *Cochrane Database of Systematic Reviews*, 1. doi:10.1002/14651858. CD005379.pub2.

Malouf, M., Grimley, E.J., & Areosa, S.A. 2008. Folic acid with or without vitamin B_{12} for cognition and dementia. *Cochrane Database of Systematic Reviews*, 4. doi:10.1002/14651858. CD004514.pub2.

McCullagh, P.J., Carswell, W., Augusto, J.C., Martin, S., Mulvenna, M.D., Zheng, H., Wang, H.Y., et al. 2009. State of the Art on Night-Time Care of People with Dementia. Paper presented at the IET Assisted Living Conference, London, March.

McGilton, K., Wells, J., Davis, A., Rochon, E., Calabrese, S., Teare, G., Naglie, G., & Biscardi, M. 2007. Rehabilitating patients with dementia who have had a hip fracture part II: Cognitive symptoms that influence care. *Topics in Geriatric Rehabilitation*, 23(2): 174–182.

National Collaborating Centre for Mental Health. 2007—Updated 2011. *Dementia: A NICE-SCIE Guideline on Supporting People with Dementia and Their Carers in Health and Social Care*. National Clinical Practice Guideline Number 42. Leicester, UK: British Psychological Society and Gaskell.

National Institute for Health and Clinical Excellence. 2011. *Dementia: Supporting People with Dementia and Their Carers in Health and Social Care*. London: NICE.

North West Joint Improvement Partnership. 2010. *Dementia Workforce Development Project: Dementia Workforce Development Mapping Report*. Droitwich, UK: Hadzor Partnership.

Parker, M., & Power, D. 2013. Management of swallowing difficulties in people with advanced dementia: Michelle Parker and Donna Power describe how a multidisciplinary approach enables best practice. *Nursing Older People*, 25(2): 26–31.

Perrin, T., & May, H. 2000. *Wellbeing in Dementia: An Occupational Approach for Therapists*. London: Churchill Livingston.

Regnier, V., & Denton, A. 2009. Ten new and emerging trends in residential group living environments. *NeuroRehabilitation*, 25: 169–188.

Scarmeas, N., Luchsinger, J., Brickman, A., Cosentino, S., Schupf, N., Xin-Tang, M., Gu, Y., & Stern, Y. 2011. Physical activity and Alzheimer's disease course. *Journal of Geriatric Psychiatry,* 19(5): 471–481.

Scheltens, P., Twisk, J.W.R., Blesa, R., Scarpini, E., von Amin, C.A.F., Bongers, A., et al. 2012. Efficacy of souvenaid in mild Alzheimer's disease: Results from a randomized, controlled trial. *Journal of Alzheimer's Disease,* 31: 225–236.

Smith, G. 2014. Light as an intervention to manage distressing symptoms in dementia: A literature review. *Mental Health Nursing,* 34(5): 12–15.

Vardy, E., & Robinson, L. 2011. Management of behavioural problems in people with dementia. *InnovAiT,* 4(6): 347–352.

Verbeek, M.H., van Rossum, E., Zwakhalen, S.M.G., Kempen, I.J.M., & Harriers, J.P.H. 2008. Small, homelike care environments for older people with dementia: A literature review. *International Psychogeriatrics,* 21(2): 252–264.

Voermans, N.C., Snijders, A.H., Schoon, Y., & Bloem, B.R. 2007. Why old people fall (and how to stop them). *Practical Neurology,* 7: 158–171.

Williamson, T. 2012. *A Stronger Collective Voice for People with Dementia.* York, UK: Joseph Roundtree Foundation.

World Health Organisation. 2010. *Global Recommendations on Physical Activity for Health.* Geneva, Switzerland: World Health Organisation.

Woods, L., Smith, G., Pendleton, J., & Parker, D. 2013. *Innovate Dementia Baseline Report: Shaping the Future for People Living with Dementia.* Liverpool, UK: Liverpool John Moores University.

Young, J., & Illsley, A. 2014. Supporting health and physical health well-being. In *Excellence in Dementia Care,* 2nd edition, edited by Downs, M., & Bowers, B., 256–270. Maidenhead, UK: Open University Press.

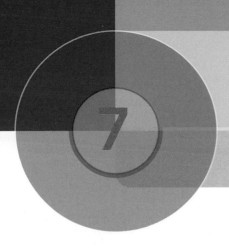

Living with dementia

CAROL WILCOCK AND TOMMY DUNNE

AIM

- To explore and consider from a personal perspective the reality of living with dementia

OBJECTIVES

- Identify the challenges and barriers to living well with dementia
- To read and learn from the narratives of a person with dementia and a carer

OVERVIEW

Living with dementia is a day-to-day challenge for both the person with dementia and the person's caregivers. There is a societal aspiration that people living with dementia can live well within their own homes, though this is based on them receiving the right support at the right time (Department of Health, 2009). The Department of Health's Dementia Strategy (2009) objective 6 aims for:

> … Provision of an appropriate range of services to support people with dementia living at home and their carers. Access to flexible and reliable services, ranging from early intervention to specialist home care services, which are responsive to the personal needs and preferences of each individual and take account of their broader family circumstances. It is accessible to people living alone or with carers, people who pay for their care privately, through personal budgets, or through local authority-arranged services. (Department of Health, 2009: 46)

This aspiration of living well with dementia is finally taking shape.

Projects are now underway across the UK with the ambition of making our communities easier places for people affected by dementia to access services, socialise and live well. Furthermore, governments are recognising the importance of wellbeing by introducing legal reforms to care across England, Wales and Northern Ireland. (Alzheimer's Society, 2014: "Executive Summary")

Certainly there is need for constant and consistent action as it is estimated that there are over 800,000 people with dementia in the UK. This figure may be an underestimation due to the issue of underdiagnosis (Woods et al., 2013; Alzheimer's Society, 2014). The challenge for society going forward is that it is predicted that the incidence of dementia will double by 2030 and more than triple by 2050 (Woods et al., 2013; World Health Organisation [WHO], 2012). Taking this into consideration, society has to ensure that the delivery of dementia care not only is fit for purpose in the here and now but also has to be flexible enough to meet this potential increase in demand (Woods et al., 2013; Alzheimer's Society, 2014; WHO, 2012). This greater emphasis on living well with dementia is a good starting place for moving forward with optimism, though there is more work to be done.

… However, the Dementia 2014 survey results indicate that still not enough has changed. Only 58% of people with dementia say they are living well, and less than half of people feel a part of their community. Approximately 40% of people felt lonely recently, and almost 10% only leave the house once a month. (Alzheimer's Society, 2014: "Executive Summary")

So what can health and social care practitioners do in the quest to help move society forward? Throughout this book a number of initiatives and practices that will help are presented, but it is also important to acknowledge that negative attitudes are, according to the Alzheimer's Society (2014) report executive summary, "'a significant barrier to people with dementia living well with the condition'. A key issue is the failure of services at times to engage meaningfully with people with dementia, which includes being respectful and listening to and acting on their needs—a *person-centred approach* (Alzheimer's Society, 2014; Kitwood, 1997).

As practitioners basing clinical judgements on professional knowledge we can sometimes forget to really listen, falling into the trap of

… reconstructing meanings to the point where an agreed true meaning is lost. (Smith, 2012: 3)

On this basis, this chapter provides an opportunity to immerse yourself in the personal stories of someone with dementia and someone who is an informal carer (Bracken & Thomas, 2005; Zeilig, 2014). When reading the narratives we want you to think about the purpose of the narrative, the content of the messages contained within the narrative, and the overall tone of the narrative and its message (Shaffer & Zikmund-Fisher, 2013). The following prompts based on the work of Shaffer and Zikmund-Fisher (2013) should be useful in your reflections; we are sure you will think of others:

Purpose
- What information is contained with the narrative?
- How does this increase your knowledge?
- How will the information assist you in engaging more effectively with people living with dementia?
- Does it prompt you to change your behaviour when caring for people with dementia?

Content
- What does the narrative say about a person's quality of life?
- How does dementia impact on their quality of life? Are there other factors present?
- Do you feel connected to their experiences? How does this make you feel?
- How does living with dementia impact on day-to-day decisions?

Tone
- Is the overall tone positive or negative?
- What factors enable a person living with dementia to feel positive?

Finally, after reflecting (Smith, 2014), consider what actions you need to take to improve your future practice.

This chapter includes two personal narratives—one from a person with dementia and one from a person who was an informal carer. Both narratives highlight the real-world challenges of living with dementia. They also give hope and inspiration.

A SERVICE USER'S NARRATIVE

I can still remember hearing those words from my psychiatrist: 'You have early-onset dementia, and it looks like Alzheimer's'. I felt my blood run cold. Did he just say I had Alzheimer's? That can't be—I'm only 58. You have to be old to get Alzheimer's, don't you?

I then thought, oh my God; my life's over, I'm going to be put in a home and have to sit in one of those chairs just staring into space without being able to speak or understand anything, a place where your family only came and visited you on birthdays and holidays.

After my dementia diagnosis, I used to hear my wife Joyce talking to her friends and family about me, but it was always in the past tense as if I had already passed away. I used to think, 'I can understand what they're talking about, so I must have been diagnosed wrong. Yeah, that's it; they've got it wrong. Everything will be all right'.

I was put on medication which included Aricept, the drug for Alzheimer's. That's when the nightmares and hallucinations really began. No one told me that these were part of the side effects of the medication or the disease. It was a lonely and scary time and one that I thought was going to be the norm for the rest of my life: 'So this is what dementia is like—family and friends avoid talking or looking at you like they used to.' I lost all confidence in myself and was frightened to talk, as I was starting to get tongue-tied when I did.

I was really down but my life started to turn around when I attended a postdiagnostic group at a local hospital, a group for people diagnosed with dementia and their family carers. It was on the last day of this group that something happened that was to have the biggest impact on my life to date. They wanted to have a service user sit on the Year of Action on Dementia (YAD) group and my wife said 'Tommy will do it'. I remember giving her a look that would have stopped a galloping horse. After all, I could hardly put two sentences together without getting tongue-tied—but I agreed to do it.

I attended the first meeting thinking to myself: 'I'm just going to be the obligatory service user name to be on the minutes just to show, "Hey look! We had a service user at the meeting"'.

The meeting started with everyone round the table introducing themselves, and everyone had important jobs. When it was my turn I said 'Tommy Dunne, service user'. You could see everyone stop, and some people were looking over their glasses at me.

Anyway, the meeting carried on with everyone saying this is what people with dementia want, and this is how they feel. I thought to myself, 'That's nothing like what people with dementia want or feel', but I didn't think I'd said it out loud. I remember it felt like the piano had stopped playing in the corner and a tumbleweed rolled up the table as everyone looked at me. The chair of the meeting said, 'Is there something you'd like to say Tommy'? I said yes, and I explained that what they had been saying about people with dementia and how we felt was nothing like what it was.

I was then given the opportunity to put my point of view over, and I could see that a few people were surprised that what I said was not what they had thought living with dementia was, and from that moment on they always asked my opinion.

Through the YAD group I got the opportunity to work with the Community Pass on the Memories Group (a local support group run by the Everton Football Club for people with dementia and their carers). There I was able to work with my peers on breaking down the stigma of dementia; it was there that I learnt a lot about carers and my peers.

I noticed that carers did all the talking for us and never gave us a chance to speak. I also noticed that carers always spoke negatively about us every time they got together. I could see that this was upsetting for my peers, so I set about getting my peers to talk about their lives and realised after hearing them that they had great stories. All of them stated that they still wanted to contribute to society but felt society would not accept them.

I also realised that family carers did not realise they were talking negatively about us on purpose because most of them were under the misapprehension that we could not understand. I also became aware that family carers needed to be able to let off steam not only for our health but also for theirs.

After a diagnosis of dementia, it became clear to me that there was no clear pathway for us or our carers; you were just left in no man's land with a feeling of total hopelessness and worse. This used to be the acceptable thing; this was accepted as normal. It was clear that something needed to be done to raise awareness of dementia and to ensure that family carers received proper training and support right from the beginning.

In the city where I live it has taken a lot of hard work and quite a few tears from all sides to get to a stage where carers are now being given the necessary training to understand the needs of a person with dementia. There are also support groups out there that carers and my peers have access to that gives us the help and support that is needed to ensure that both carers and my peers are able to live well with dementia, but there is a lot more to be done.

If ever I needed proof that people were now listening to us people with dementia, the proof came in 2013 when I was awarded the Merseycare NHS Positive Achievement Award and the Winner of Winners award. This was a proud day for me as I felt that I had helped break down the stigma of dementia and showed that we could contribute to society.

My goal now in life is to ensure that people with dementia are diagnosed earlier and are shown that there is nothing to fear and that with the right support they and their families can live well with dementia. After all, we do not live in the past or the future. We live in the present, and it is called the present for a reason—because the greatest gift you can give someone is your time because when you dedicate your time you are offering a part of your life that you will never get back.

A CARER'S NARRATIVE

In the summer of 2003 I retired from teaching. My husband Terry had retired from his work as a mechanical engineer 3 years previously. We had gone through the usual stages in our lives together: meeting and falling in love, marriage, setting up home, developing our respective careers, having children and sharing interests. We were now looking forward to enjoying our retirement years. We were able to celebrate our ruby wedding anniversary, but this stage of our lives together was to be cut short by the onset in Terry of both Parkinson's and Alzheimer's.

For 2 years nothing much changed but looking back, there were telltale signs there which at the time did not seem especially significant, or maybe I just chose to ignore them and push them to the back of my mind. For example, there was an increasing tendency to repeat things, an impairment in the driving skills of someone who had been an excellent driver, and a deterioration in sense of direction when in a new environment. Perhaps most upsetting was the increasing difficulty in performing do-it-yourself tasks for someone who had always been able to tackle any job with ease.

As 2005 progressed, other problems had become apparent. By now I was doing all the driving and Terry was experiencing difficulties with some aspects of dressing. Tying shoelaces, fastening a tie and even putting on a sweater posed problems. The shoelaces problem was an easy one to solve by buying shoes with Velcro fasteners.

By the end of 2005 there was a marked deterioration in Terry's condition. Understandably, he became depressed at times as he was aware that something was wrong. Problems with dressing increased and also difficulties with climbing steps and changing direction at the top of the stairs began to develop. At this point neither of us could ignore what was happening so we went together to see our general practitioner (GP), who had no hesitation in referring Terry to a consultant in old age psychiatry who did various tests and sent Terry for a brain scan. In 2006 a formal diagnosis of Alzheimer's and Parkinson's was made, medication was prescribed and regular check ups with the consultant were put in place. In truth, the diagnosis, though devastating, was a confirmation of what I already knew, or at least suspected, and I should probably have sought medical advice earlier. I know that some carers feel let down with the professional advice and care they receive, but I cannot speak too highly of the consultant, who was always prepared to spend time listening to my concerns and most important, was always honest with me about the progression of the illness.

Dementia sufferers often lose any sense of connection to previous relationships and activities, so after the formal diagnosis I made a conscious decision to try, as far as possible, to carry on as normal. I tried to focus not only on managing Terry's symptoms but also on Terry the person so that we continued doing the sorts of activities he had always enjoyed and I was determined he was going to get pleasure from for as long as possible. We had always enjoyed holidays in Italy but after our visit there in 2006 I realised that airport procedures and being in such a different environment were distressing for Terry, so we adapted to having short breaks in England, particularly in the Lake District which he had always loved since biking holidays there as a teenager. We also went on day trips to Liverpool, Southport and Chester, making good use of our free rail passes. We renewed our season tickets for St Helens Rugby League and attended all the home matches plus two Grand Finals at Old Trafford. Terry's attention might have wandered somewhat in the second half, but he really looked forward to going, and this more than compensated for any difficulties encountered in negotiating the turnstiles and the steps up to our seats.

Although receiving a confirmation of dementia is a devastating blow, I firmly believe that there can still be happiness after diagnosis. Those with the illness are still themselves inside and they can continue to love and enjoy what they used to take pleasure from before the illness. Communication is so important; those with dementia might not always be able to articulate what they are feeling but they feel nonetheless, and words and gestures of encouragement are therefore so important. Touch is a fundamental human need, and the simple act of holding a hand can give comfort, reassurance and pleasure.

Until the middle of 2008, the deterioration in Terry's condition was a gradual one, but suddenly in the summer of that year a marked change occurred. There was disturbed sleep for both of us and I felt increasingly uneasy about leaving him on his own. On one occasion he wandered off and although fortunately he hadn't gone far, that 30 minutes until I found him seemed like forever. Terry started to need more and more help with dressing and eating, and he became increasingly unsteady on his feet. I had to make myself be patient and try not to rush things along, but this was sometimes easier said than done, especially when combined with a lack of sleep. Sometimes Terry didn't recognise me and kept asking to go home. This was obviously distressing for me but I came to realise that it must have been even more frightening and distressing for him. I was reminded of lines written in the nineteenth century by the poet John Clare, who suffered from a mental illness:

> Even the dearest, that I love the best
> Are strange—nay rather stranger than the rest.

I will never forget the look of sheer relief on Terry's face when, after some reassurance, he realised who I was and the world made sense to him again.

With the help of a loving and supportive family, my two daughters and Terry's brother and sister, I was able to cope with the situation. I also used the service provided by Crossroads Care (an organisation which provides support for carers in their homes). One of their staff would stay with Terry if I needed to go out when no family member was available. Everything changed, however, when physical aggression toward me, especially at night, started to become a frequent occurrence. This was so unlike the Terry I had always known, who was a kind and gentle person, and was a really frightening experience when I feared for his safety as well as my own.

The consultant, having seen Terry and talked with me, advised that the time had come for Terry to be admitted to an assessment ward. I knew at this point that it was the right and inevitable step. I will never forget the day Terry went in. Seeing him walk away from us down the corridor was a defining moment for me, our two daughters, Clare and Jane, and Terry's brother Stan.

The ward was under the management of a nurse manager who was a strong advocate of person-centred care. This was a philosophy followed by her staff so that the care Terry received during his 4 months as a patient and the support I was given were excellent. We cannot care for someone unless we care about them, and we cannot care about them unless we know who they are. I was so fortunate that when I was no longer caring for Terry at home, those who took on that responsibility were so committed to their role. They treated him with respect and never forgot that he was an individual, taking time to find out about his life, his background, career and interests. Memories are so important as they give us a sense of self, something to hold on to and make sense of the world around us.

Little things are so important when you entrust a loved one to someone else's care. I will always remember leaving one day after visiting and when I looked into the lounge, one of the staff was sitting with Terry and stroking his hand. On another occasion, another staff member told me that the previous evening she had been playing music for the patients and that although Terry could not get up and dance, he had been tapping his foot. One of the male staff, himself a keen Saints (St Helens Rugby League) supporter and knowing that Terry was, too, often used to talk to him about the team. Little things do mean a lot.

At visiting time on the ward I got to talk to other carers who were in the same position as I was. I hadn't gone to any carer support groups when Terry was at home, which would probably have helped me as, when I used to look around, everyone else appeared to be living normal lives and I seemed to be the only one caring for someone with dementia.

In the spring of 2009 Terry's condition began to deteriorate rapidly. He was experiencing difficulty swallowing and developed a series of chest infections. At the age of just 68, Terry died peacefully of pneumonia and a collapsed lung on April 15 in hospital, with me, his daughters Clare and Jane, and brother Stan around him.

Dementia is a cruel illness, both for the person who has it and for the carers, families and friends who witness it. Grief does not end but I have tried to come to terms with it and to get something positive from what was a devastating experience. I did this firstly by becoming a carer support volunteer on the assessment ward and now as a trustee of the Hargreaves Dementia Trust, a local charity based in St Helens.

Those with dementia are people just like you and me. What has happened to them could happen to any one of us, irrespective of our background or intelligence. If it does then we have to hope that there will be someone there, as there was for Terry, to hold our hand, to preserve that thread of humanity, to give us that person-centred care and to treat us with respect.

CHAPTER SUMMARY

Living well with dementia is a societal aspiration; this is based on those with dementia receiving the right support at the right time.

Negative attitudes can be a significant barrier to people with dementia living well with the condition.

As practitioners basing clinical judgements on professional knowledge we can sometimes forget to really listen to people living with dementia, therefore it is important to think about the purpose of their narrative, the content of the messages contained within their narrative, and the overall tone of their narrative.

People living with dementia can contribute positively to society and as practitioners we always need to deliver care that is respectful and person centred.

REFLECTION ON LEARNING

1. What is the societal aspiration for people living with dementia?
2. What does the Department of Health's Dementia Strategy (2009) objective 6 aim to do?
3. Why is the figure of over 800,000 people with dementia potentially an underestimation?
4. In terms of people diagnosed with dementia, what is the challenge for society going forward?
5. According to the Alzheimer's Society (2014) report what is the significant barrier to people with dementia living well with the condition?
6. When listening to people living with dementia what trap can practitioners fall into?
7. When listening to and thinking about the narrative of a person living with dementia, what is useful to consider?
8. What does it feel like to be diagnosed with dementia?
9. What are the day-to-day challenges of living with dementia? Also identify potential solutions.
10. Why is person-centred care so important?

REFERENCES

Alzheimer's Society. 2014. *Dementia UK*, 2nd edition. London: Alzheimer's Society.

Bracken, P., & Thomas, P. 2005. *Postpsychiatry: Mental Health in a Postmodern World*. Oxford, UK: Oxford University Press.

Department of Health. 2009. *Living Well with Dementia: A National Dementia Strategy*. London: Department of Health.

Kitwood, T. 1997. *Dementia Reconsidered*. London: Open University Press.

Shaffer, V.A., & Zikmund-Fisher, B.J. 2013. All stories are not alike: A purpose-, content-, and valence-based taxonomy of patient narratives in decision aids. *Medical Decision Making*, 33: 4–13.

Smith, G. 2012. An introduction to psychological interventions. In *Psychological Interventions in Mental Health Nursing*, edited by Smith, G., 1–10. Maidenhead, UK: Open University Press.

Smith, G. 2014. *Mental Health Nursing at a Glance*. Chichester, UK: Wiley Blackwell.

Woods, L., Smith, G., Pendleton, J., & Parker, D. 2013. *Innovate Dementia Baseline Report: Shaping the Future for People Living with Dementia*. Liverpool, UK: Liverpool John Moores University.

World Health Organisation. 2012. *Dementia: A Public Health Priority*. Geneva, Switzerland: World Health Organisation.

Zeilig, H. 2014. Dementia as a cultural metaphor. *The Gerontologist*, 54(2): 258–267.

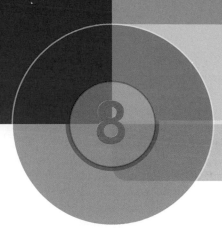

Care and compassion

8

JULIE ANN HAYES, LORRAINE SHAW, AND
GRAHAME SMITH

AIM

- To appreciate the compassionate care of people living with dementia within an ethical context

OBJECTIVES

- To discuss ethical practice and its relationship to ethical reasoning
- To explore the ethical underpinnings of a person-centred approach
- To reflect on the use of a value-based approach
- To consider the human rights and autonomy of a person diagnosed with dementia

OVERVIEW

The aim of this chapter is to explore the compassionate care of people living with dementia. The report of the Mid Staffordshire NHS Foundation Trust Public Inquiry—Executive Summary (Francis, 2013) is clear that care delivery should be compassionate. Taking a normative position that nurses should deliver compassionate care places compassion as a care issue within an ethical context (Francis, 2013; Smith, 2012c). Taking this into consideration this chapter frames compassionate care as an ethical issue and in doing so explores the potential ethical challenges the nurse may encounter. Further, there is the expectation that people with dementia not only will receive compassionate care but also are actively supported to live well with dementia. The Department of Health's (DH) (2009) national dementia strategy makes the point that 'positive input from health and social care services can make all the difference between living well with dementia and having a poor quality of life' (p. 7).

Nurses are professionally expected to act ethically and 'do the right thing'—in this case, deliver compassionate care (Nursing and Midwifery Council [NMC], 2015). The NMC's revised professional code (2015), updated from 2008, now uses the term *compassion* with the expectation that the nurse will 'treat people with kindness, respect and compassion' (p. 4), and that 'when people are in distress the nurse will respond compassionately and kindly' (p. 5). Being ethical is not just about following the rules; the NMC's professional code does not provide a set of rules that will assist the nurse to resolve every ethical dilemma the nurse faces within his or her practice (Smith, 2012c). Rather it provides a framework that will assist the nurse to be more effective when ethically reasoning through these day-to-day practice challenges (Ford, 2006; Smith, 2012c; NMC, 2015). This chapter examines the 'rules' in more detail. It provides a balanced approach, accepting that to act ethically the nurse has to consider the role values play when delivering care (Fulford, 2009; Smith, 2012c). Values are evident in dementia care, especially where practice has a controlling element, such as managing clinical risk, with the outcome that certain freedoms are restricted by the same nurse who is also expected to deliver compassionate care (Smith, 2012c; Fulford, 2009). The ability to work with values that are inherent within a given situation enables the nurse to safeguard the person with dementia in a way that will reduce the potential abuse of this power to control (Smith, 2012c; Chodoff, 2009; Woodbridge & Fulford, 2004; Francis, 2013).

This process of being ethical, working with rules and values, does not happen in a vacuum. Being ethical and delivering compassionate care are based on the nurse being an effective communicator (Smith, 2014). It is also important that the nurse recognises that within a dementia care context the therapeutic relationship is a medium for treatment, especially when delivering psychological interventions (Smith, 2012b, 2014; NMC, 2010). Let us consider the following chapter scenario which shapes our journey through this chapter:

Molly, an elderly patient with dementia who is unable to walk due to severe osteoarthritis, persists in getting out of bed unaided during the night and repeatedly falls to the floor. Due to the layout of the ward and the lack of staff, constant observation is not possible. Helen, the registered nurse, begins her night shift and is in charge of the unit and the care of Molly. She had cared for Molly earlier in the week, and during the night two incident forms had to be completed due to Molly's falls. There is a lack of staff due to sickness, and Helen is working with members of staff who are not familiar with the unit. Helen is aware that additional sedation is not recommended for Molly as it has affected her response to treatment, but Helen is also aware that it is unsafe to leave Molly considering her previous falls. Helen is anxious about the night ahead and contemplates if she should contact the medical team to prescribe additional sedation for Molly.

BEING ETHICAL

To act ethically a nurse must be adept at ethical reasoning, which includes being able to systematically select and utilise a relevant ethical theory (Smith, 2012c; Bloch & Green, 2009; Barker 2011). In essence, ethical theories can be divided into normative and non-normative theories. This section concentrates on normative theories (Sumner, 1967; Smith, 2012c). These theories relate to the pursuit of describing what actions are right or wrong, what ought to be done or not done, what motives are good or bad, and what characteristics are virtuous (Smith, 2012c; Barker, 2011).

Consequentialism or utilitarianism as an ethical theory takes the general view that whether an action is ethical or not ethical is determined by the outcome of that action. To be ethical, a nurse's action should 'produce the greatest balance of good over bad' (Smith, 2012c; Bloch & Green, 2009). Whereas deontology, or Kantianism, focuses on duties rather than outcomes, the ethical nurse without exception must always do his or her duty (e.g. not to lie or steal) (Smith, 12012c; LaFollette, 2000). In virtue ethics, a nurse must be virtuous. This requires the nurse to develop specific character traits such as honesty and trustworthiness (Smith & Godfrey, 2002; Smith, 2012c). Care ethics, building on virtue ethics, values the context of care with an emphasis on promoting the well-being of those who give care and those who receive care. On this basis the delivery of compassionate care would be seen as being ethical care (Bloch & Green, 2009; Horsfall et al., 2011; Smith, 2012c). Principlism is less of an ethical theory and more of an ethical reasoning approach. As its name suggests, it is principle based, and according to this approach the ethical nurse would base his or her decision-making on the following principles: do no harm (non-maleficence); act to benefit others (beneficence); respect a person's autonomy; and treat people fairly (justice) (Beauchamp & Childress, 2009; Barker, 2011; Smith, 2012c).

Being adept at ethical reasoning also means nurses need to know which ethical rules they should be adhering to. This will include professional and legal frameworks, policies, and clinical guidelines (Smith, 2012c; Mitchell, 2011; Callaghan, 2009). The nurse as a registered professional will also be expected to act in a certain way, adhering to expected professional standards, behaviours, and values. In other words, nurses will have to comply with the NMC's (2015) code of professional conduct. When resolving ethical dilemmas the code, like other ethical rules, provides the nurse with a point of reference for shaping their ethical reasoning (Smith, 2012c; Ford, 2006; NMC, 2015).

As discussed so far, being adept at ethical reasoning requires the nurse to be able to identify the relevant ethical theory and understand and reference the 'rules'. In addition the nurse will need to be able to identify an ethical issue, such as in the case of the scenario of 'prescribing of additional sedation', and then critically reflect on those identified issues in a rational and systematic way (Fulford, Thornton, & Graham, 2006; Smith, 2012c; Ford, 2006). This process, based on the work of Smith (2012c: 148), would look something like the following:

1. Recognise the ethical issue(s)
2. Gather the facts and examine values
3. Consider the rules
4. Look at any underpinning moral theories
5. Consider all options
6. Make a decision and test it
7. Act and reflect on the outcome

Returning to the scenario, when considering the ethical responses to the scenario, let us consider what impact ethical theory might have:

Firstly, the utilitarian perspective may suggest the right action is to sedate Molly, the consequences of this being the greater balance of good over bad in relation to maximising the care resources for the other patients. Taking the deontological approach, it would be unacceptable to sedate Molly as this would not be acting in accordance with duty; also, sedating Molly would be using her as a means to another end (i.e. maximising care for others at the cost of Molly's own needs). Both virtue ethics and care ethics would require the nurse not to sedate Molly; the value placed on each individual and the individual's care needs outweighs taking into account the needs of others. Using principlism would encourage the nurse to reason, taking into account possible benefits, harms, and Molly's right to autonomy and just treatment. Again, the outcome would be not to sedate; as Molly lacks capacity to make an autonomous decision, the nurse must act as her advocate. It is clear the benefits of not sedating outweigh the harms, and Molly has a right to adequate care as do all other people on the ward.

A PERSON-CENTRED APPROACH

A person-centred approach to the planning and delivery of care for people living with dementia is fundamental, with all parties involved in the process being viewed as equal partners (Parker, 2012; Woods et al., 2013). This approach should draw on the skills and knowledge of people living with dementia in a way that they are viewed as experts in their own care (Parker, 2012; Mast, 2014). In addition, a person-centred approach will aim to safeguard the human value and individuality of a person with dementia. It is holistic and looks at the whole of the person, including taking into account the person's social and support networks, and it prioritises the person's perspective with a focus on promoting well-being (Parker, 2012; Mast, 2014; Kitwood, 1997).

Nurses as professionals are required to engage in and promote person-centred care; it must be compassionate and empowering. To do this they need to be effective communicators (NMC, 2015; Francis, 2013; Commissioning Board, 2012; Knott, 2012). To be effective communicators, those in nursing must be self-aware, they must have the necessary communication skills, and they must also recognise that communication as a process is two-way, with information constantly shared and processed by all involved parties (Knott, 2012). Communication can be broken down into non-verbal and verbal communication; non-verbal communication involves utilising and paying attention to

- Facial expressions
- Eye contact
- Gestures
- Posture
- Head movements
- Personal space
- Touch
- Appearance (Smith, 2014: 3)

Verbal communication is not only the words we use but also includes the way the spoken word is conveyed (paralanguage) and the way the spoken word is perceived by the other person (meta-communication) (Knott, 2012). While communicating, the nurse will also need to actively listen to what is being said and then will need to respond in a way that is appropriate for the situation (Knott, 2012). Nurses will also have to be aware, for example, that people living with dementia are potentially at their most vulnerable during the care process; therefore it is essential that the nurse is empathetic (Smith, 2014). In conjunction, the nurse will be expected to demonstrate the following values and behaviours (the 6 Cs):

Care – people receiving care expect it to be right for them, throughout every stage of their life

Compassion – can also be described as intelligent kindness, and is central to how people perceive their care

Competence – having the expertise, clinical and technical knowledge to deliver effective care

Communication – is central to successful caring relationships and to effective team working

Courage – enables us to do the right thing for the people we care for, to speak up when we have concerns

Commitment – to our patients and populations is a cornerstone of what we do
(Commissioning Board, 2012: 13)

The communication process does not exist within a vacuum. It will be a crucial part of building and sustaining a therapeutic relationship, one that is based on the delivery of safe and effective care (Perraud et al., 2006; Smith, 2012b). As mentioned previously it is essential that the nurse, as an effective communicator, within this relationship is empathetic; this includes being able to be

- An active listener
- Genuinely interested
- Accepting of the person
- Caring and compassionate (Smith, 2014: 5)

Key to a nurse building a sustainable therapeutic relationship that is meaningful and positive is not only about empathy but also skill in the therapeutic and ethical use of self (Smith, 2012b; Martinez, 2009). This includes

- Selecting the right words to use
- Knowing when to talk and when to be silent
- Using the right verbal and non-verbal responses
- Adapting non-verbal communication to suit the situation (Smith, 2014: 5)

Part of engendering expertise in the therapeutic use of self is the nurse's expert use of critical reflection, which

> … is a process which requires the … nurse to not only re-examine their practice experiences, but also to focus on changing their practice for the better, meaning that they need to action plan and then act upon this plan. (Smith, 2012a: 160)

By expertly reflecting, the nurse will develop a seamless understanding of the impact their self has on others and they will be able to use this knowledge in a way changes their practice for the betterment of people in their care (Smith, 2012a, 2014). Now let us return to the scenario and consider the impact that being person centred can have on the care of Molly:

Person-centred care in this context would require the nurse to tailor Molly's care to Molly's specific needs, to consider her point of view, and to reflect critically on the dilemma. The outcome would be not to sedate. In addition it would require the nurse to review Molly's care plan to see if it is truly person centred and has included the input of the family/carer and directs staff to Molly's specific needs.

VALUE-BASED PRACTICE

Adept ethical reasoning is structured; it is also situated in the real-time decisions that the nurses make in their everyday practice. It is underpinned by person centeredness (Smith, 2012a). The implication is that to be effective in their ethical reasoning endeavours nurses must work with the facts, and they must also work with the inherent values (Smith, 2012c; Fulford, 2009; Ford, 2006). Thinking ethically within the field of dementia brings its own unique challenges. One of those challenges is the complex use of power; as an example, within the field of dementia there are times when a person with dementia can be treated without his or her consent (Smith, 2012c). Given the complexity of caring for the person with dementia and the emphasis on risk management, it is all too common for this issue of power to be overlooked (Smith, 2012c).

Overlooking the issue of power can arise from the assumption that assigning a diagnosis of dementia, knowing when a person with dementia lacks capacity, and being able to predict risk are clear and objective judgements (Roberts, 2004; Fulford, 2009; Smith, 2012c). The use of assessment frameworks and tools helps justify these judgements, but ultimately this process is dependent on a person with the person's unique perspective weighing the evidence and making a decision, one that cannot be totally divorced from any inherent values (Fulford, 2009). A nurse may feel at a personal level compelled to protect a person living with dementia; this may in turn lead to the nurse being cautious about the way he or she manages risk, in turn influencing the nurse not to take positive risks even if the person within his or her care prefers that approach.

Going back to the ethical reasoning process and looking at using facts, we have to acknowledge that facts and values are intertwined (Smith, 2012c). This also feeds into the use of moral theory; for example, principlism provides a rational and a reasoned approach to processing ethical issues but it has its limits, especially when dealing with complex and real-time issues, such as fluctuating capacity. One nurse may determine at a given moment in time that a person with dementia has capacity, but another nurse does not; an agreed assessment tool may help to resolve the disagreement in part, but capacity can fluctuate minute to minute (Beauchamp & Childress, 2009; Fulford, 2009; Bolmsjo, Sandman, & Andersson, 2006). The challenge is that nurses need to effectively deal with these types of scenarios on a regular basis; they also need to be aware that an on-the-spot judgement is more likely to be value based (Smith, 2012c). So how do we make sense of values in a way that is ethical? Value-based practice enables the nurse to sensitively pay attention to the value-laden nature of their practice through focusing not on outcomes but on following a good process (Woodbridge & Fulford, 2004; Fulford, 2009; Smith, 2012c). The nurse should

1. Consider the perspective of the person with dementia: What does the person want?
2. Take a balanced approach; equally consider the person's perspective as well as the rules.
3. Make sure the person's story is not lost in the language of science and professionalism.
4. Always listen actively to the person.

We now return to Molly:

A diagnosis of dementia does not mean a person is automatically lacking capacity; however judgements to the contrary can be all too prevalent. In Molly's case her state of confusion does suggest limited capacity, however not being able to consent to taking sedation does not give a nurse the legitimate right to administer sedation as this action would be difficult to justify given the potential harms that could result.

HUMAN RIGHTS

Balancing values and facts, being person centred, and continually referencing the rules is a challenge for the nurse, especially if a person with dementia lacks capacity (Thompson et al., 2006; Callaghan, 2009; Roberts, 2005). In this situation the nurse is sanctioned by society to act on behalf of the individual; in some cases when the level of risk is high the nurse will be expected to exert control (Roberts, 2004, 2005). The added dimension to this use of control is that society expects this sanctioned power to be based on 'objectivity':

> The concern is that ethical objectivity may be seen as sure defence against the abuse in the field of mental health, but if we accept the value-laden nature of the mental health field then abuse can be seen as a real and present danger and potentially a major ethical issue. (Smith, 2012c: 151)

By being person-centred and reflecting constantly on his or her practice, the nurse will ensure that the use of this power will not be hidden away (Smith, 2012c, 2014). To support this way of working, there are a number of legal frameworks in which the nurse must structure his or her practice; the added benefit of these frameworks is that they protect the rights of people with dementia (Smith, 2014). These frameworks include the Mental Health Act (MHA) 1983 of England and Wales, amended by the MHA 2007; Mental Capacity Act (MCA) 2005 (DH, 2005), applying to England and Wales; and the Human Rights Act 1998, which came into full force in the UK in 2000 (Smith, 2014). In this section we explore the Human Rights Act in more detail. This act focuses on protecting the rights of individuals, and these rights are reflected through a number of articles. The articles particularly relevant to people with dementia are the right to life (Article 2), the prohibition of torture (Article 3), the right to liberty and security (Article 5), and the right to respect for private and family life (Article 8) (Smith, 2014). Let us look at how this relates to Molly:

When we are considering the case of Molly, the articles in the Human Rights Act that present a challenge for a nurse are Articles 3 and 5. If the nurse were to consider not sedating Molly in this scenario and allowing the risk of falls and potentially further harm, then would this equate to torture? Arguably, the issue 'to not treat' constitutes torture has been rejected in a number of cases (Hoppe & Miola, 2014).

Article 5, the right to liberty and security, presents many issues for the nurse in this scenario. If we agree that Molly lacks capacity due to serious mental health illness of dementia, then we can assume that the nurse will be treating Molly using the principle of 'best interests' and considering the 'least-restrictive' option (anything done for or on behalf of a person who lacks capacity should be least restrictive of their basic rights and freedoms).

The health-care team may employ the 'deprivation of liberty' safeguards as part of the MCA of 2005. The safeguards should ensure that a care home, hospital or supported living arrangement only deprives someone of liberty in a safe and correct way, and that this is only done when it is in the best interests of the person and there is no other way to look after the person.

AUTONOMY

The principle of respect for autonomy requires respect for the choice made by an individual. In the context of healthcare, the patient has a right to decide for himself or herself. Autonomy refers to the capacity of an individual to make an informed and independent decision about their care. The MHA (1983/2007) of England and Wales is a legal framework under which a person with dementia can be compulsorily admitted, detained and treated in hospital (Smith, 2014). It has a number of sections which detail what it is and is not allowed under the act. Some of these sections allow a person detained under the act to be treated without his or her consent (Smith, 2014).

A key factor in determining treatment without consent is capacity; if a person lacks capacity this is sometimes described as being non-autonomous (Smith, 2012c). To be autonomous means to be able to choose for oneself; this is often viewed as self-determination and self-governance (Buka, 2015). Self-determination involves individuals being able to formulate and carry out their own plans and wishes; self-governance extends and implies that individuals are able to govern their own lives by rules and values (Buka, 2015). Both self-determination and self-governance are dependent on the person having both the mental and the physical capacity to make choices and decisions and the ability to put them into action (Buka, 2015).

In relation to the MCA of 2005, individuals are determined to have capacity to make their own decisions on the basis that they can

- Understand information relevant to the decision
- Retain, use and weigh that information in the process of making that decision
- Communicate that decision (Smith, 2014: 63)

Where individuals are deemed to lack capacity the MCA of 2005 provides a supportive and transparent process. Here, it is important to recognise that a lack of capacity can be both temporary and transient (Smith, 2014). Returning to Molly's situation, let us consider how the act could be used:

The scenario surrounding Molly provides the nurse with some challenging considerations. If we consider autonomy, the competent patient has the right to refuse any form of medical intervention, therefore we respect the patient's right to self-rule and self-determine. In the case of Molly, this differs somewhat; the effects of a serious mental health illness such as dementia on the levels of competence will render Molly incapable of making a competent decision regarding her care. The MCA of 2005 provides measures to support the nurse to promote autonomy, although patient capacity is lost.

These measures are as follows:

- Individuals being supported to make their own decisions: All practicable help must be given before anyone is treated as not being able to make their own decisions. This would take the format of advocates. These advocates could be personal advocates such as those with lasting power of attorney, legal advocates, or independent mental capacity advocates.

- Best interests: An act done or decision made under the act for or on behalf of a person who lacks capacity must be done in the person's best interests. Contained within the act is a comprehensive checklist of factors to be taken into account by decision-makers when making decisions about best interests of a patient who lacks capacity.

CHAPTER SUMMARY

Nurses must be adept at ethical reasoning, which is a structured process; during this process, the nurse must be able to select and utilise a relevant ethical theory.

Being ethical is also about being person centred; to be person centred, the nurse should draw on the skills and knowledge of people living with dementia in a way that they are viewed as experts in their own care.

Ethical reasoning as a structure is not a recipe to be strictly adhered to; it must also pay attention to the valued-laden nature of dementia care.

To balance the sanctioned power that society gives to the nurse, nurses must understand that people with dementia have rights and freedoms and these rights are protected by a number of legal frameworks.

REFLECTION ON LEARNING

1. Define the ethical theory of deontology.
2. Consequentialism, also known as utilitarianism, generally takes the view that determining whether an action is ethical or not ethical is based on the outcome of that action: What are the implications for the mental health nurse caring for Molly?
3. What is principlism?
4. What does the concept of capacity mean?
5. Define the term *autonomy*.
6. What are the means by which a registered nurse (RN) enables the patient to be autonomous?
7. The notion of best interests is defined within the MCA (2005). What does best interests mean?
8. What is the role of a lasting power of attorney?
9. What is the role of an independent mental capacity advocate?
10. Within the MCA (2005) the health team may employ the 'deprivation of liberty' safeguards. What do these safeguards mean, and who can they be applied to?

REFERENCES

Barker, P. 2011. Ethics: In search of the good life. In *Mental Health Ethics: The Human Context*, edited by Barker, P., 5–30. London: Routledge.

Beauchamp, T.L., & Childress, J.F. 2009. *Principles of Biomedical Ethics*, 6th edition. Oxford, UK: Oxford University Press.

Bloch, S., & Green, S.A. 2009. The scope of psychiatric ethics. In *Psychiatric Ethics*, 4th edition, edited by Bloch, S., & Green, S.A., 3–8. Oxford, UK: Oxford University Press.

Bolmsjo, I.A., Sandman, L., & Andersson, E. 2006. Everyday ethics in the care of elderly people. *Nursing Ethics*, 3(3): 249–263.

Buka, P. 2015. *Patients' Rights, Law and Ethics for Nurses*, 2nd edition. Boca Raton, FL: CRC Press.

Callaghan, P. 2009. Introduction: Mental nursing past, present, and future. In *Mental Health Nursing Skills*, edited by Callaghan, P., Playle, J., & Cooper, L., 2–9. Oxford, UK: Oxford University Press.

Chodoff, P. 2009. The abuse of psychiatry. In *Psychiatric Ethics*, 4th edition, edited by Bloch, S., & Green, S.A., 99–110. Oxford, UK: Oxford University Press.

Commissioning Board: Chief Nursing Officer and DH Chief Nursing Adviser. 2012. *Compassion in Practice*. London: DH and the NHS Commissioning Board.

Department of Health (1983). *Mental Health Act*. London: HMSO.

Department of Health. 2005. *Mental Capacity Act*. London: HMSO.

Department of Health. 2009. *Living Well with Dementia: A National Dementia Strategy*. London: Department of Health.

Ford, G.G. 2006. *Ethical Reasoning for Mental Health Professionals*. London: Sage.

Francis, R. 2013. *Report of the Mid Staffordshire NHS Foundation Trust Public Inquiry— Executive Summary*. London: Stationery Office.

Fulford, K.W.M. 2009. Values, science and psychiatry. In *Psychiatric Ethics*, 4th edition, edited by Bloch, S., & Green, S.A., 61–84. Oxford, UK: Oxford University Press.

Fulford, K.W.M., Thornton, T., & Graham, G. 2006. *Oxford Textbook of Philosophy and Psychiatry*. Oxford, UK: Oxford University Press.

Hoppe, N., & Miola, J. 2014. *Medical Law and Medical Ethics*. Cambridge, UK: Cambridge University Press.

Horsfall, J., Cleary, M., Hunt, G.E., & Walter, G. 2011. Acute care. In *Mental Health Ethics: The Human Context*, edited by Barker, P., 197–204. London: Routledge.

Kitwood, T. 1997. *Dementia Reconsidered*. London: Open University Press.

Knott, D. 2012. From communication skills to psychological interventions. In *Psychological Interventions*, edited by Smith, G., 24–36. Maidenhead, UK: Open University Press.

LaFollette, H. 2000. Introduction. In *The Blackwell Guide to Ethical Theory*, edited by LaFollette, H., 1–12. Oxford, UK: Blackwell.

Martinez, R. 2009. Narrative ethics. In *Psychiatric Ethics*, 4th edition, edited by Bloch, S., & Green, S.A., 49–60. Oxford, UK: Oxford University Press.

Mast, B. 2014. Whole person assessment and care planning. In *Excellence in Dementia Care*, 2nd edition, edited by Downs, M., & Bowers, B., 290–302. Maidenhead, UK: Open University Press.

Mitchell, V. 2011. Professional relationships. In *Mental Health Ethics: The Human Context*, edited by Barker, P., 149–158. London: Routledge.

Nursing and Midwifery Council. 2010. *Standards for Pre-registration Nursing Education*. London: Nursing and Midwifery Council.

Nursing and Midwifery Council. 2015. *The Code: Professional Standards of Practice and Behaviour for Nurses and Midwives*. London: Nursing and Midwifery Council.

Parker, D. 2012. Psychological interventions and working with the older adult. In *Psychological Interventions*, edited by Smith, G., 120–131. Maidenhead, UK: Open University Press.

Perraud, S., Delaney, K.R., Carlson-Sabelli, L., Johnson, M.E., Shephard, R., & Paun, O. 2006. Advanced practice psychiatric mental health nursing, finding our core: The therapeutic relationship in 21st century. *Perspectives in Psychiatric Care*, 42(4): 215–226.

Roberts, M. 2004. Psychiatric ethics: A critical introduction for mental health nurses. *Journal of Psychiatric and Mental Health Nursing*, 11: 583–588.

Roberts, M. 2005. The production of the psychiatric subject: Power, knowledge and Michel Foucault. *Nursing Philosophy*, 6: 33–42.

Smith, G. 2012a. Conclusion: Psychological interventions and the mental health nurse's future development. In *Psychological Interventions*, edited by Smith, G., 155–164. Maidenhead, UK: Open University Press.

Smith, G. 2012b. An introduction to psychological interventions. In *Psychological Interventions*, edited by Smith, G., 1–10. Maidenhead, UK: Open University Press.

Smith, G. 2012c. Psychological interventions within an ethical context. In *Psychological Interventions*, edited by Smith, G., 143–154. Maidenhead, UK: Open University Press.

Smith, G. 2014. *Mental Health Nursing at a Glance*. Chichester, UK: Wiley Blackwell.

Smith, K.V., & Godfrey, N.S. 2002. Being a good nurse and doing the right thing: A qualitative study. *Nursing Ethics*, 9(3): 301–312.

Sumner, L.W. 1967. Normative ethics and metaethics. *Ethics*, 77(2): 95–106.

Thompson, I.E, Melia, K.M., Boyd, K.M., & Horsburgh, D. 2006. *Nursing Ethics*, 5th edition. London: Churchill Livingston.

Woodbridge, K., & Fulford, K.W.M. 2004. *Whose Values? A Workbook for Values-Based Practice in Mental Health Care*. London: Sainsbury Centre for Mental Health.

Woods, L., Smith, G., Pendleton, J., & Parker, D. 2013. *Innovate Dementia Baseline Report: Shaping the Future for People Living with Dementia*. Liverpool, UK: Liverpool John Moores University.

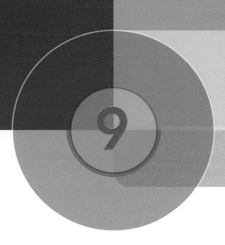

Pharmacological interventions

9

REBECCA RYLANCE AND DONAL DEEHAN

AIM

- To provide an overview of the current medication options along with the best practice principles in relation to medicine management for people who live with dementia

OBJECTIVES

- To identify the key principles of medicine management and the 'five rights of drug administration'
- To discuss the recommended treatments for mild to moderate Alzheimer's disease and the relevant national guidelines
- To identify how pain is assessed amongst people who live with dementia
- To examine the best practice principles of non-medical prescribing

OVERVIEW

This chapter examines the best practice principles of pharmacological assessment, medicine management and prescribing. The chapter also discusses the safe administration of medicines and the relevant legislation and codes which govern best practice. A clinical scenario is used throughout the chapter to underpin the key learnings. The scenario follows the journey of 'Ellen'. As you read the chapter, think about Ellen and how the principles of medication management can be applied. The chapter discusses the licensed pharmacological agents for the cognitive symptoms of dementia. It also discusses some of the pharmacotherapies for non-cognitive symptoms. The issue of pain management in the context of Ellen also is examined and how the assessment of pain may differ for a person living with dementia who may be experiencing cognitive impairment. The chapter concludes with a short 'self-assessment' quiz which will help consolidate your learning.

MEDICATION MANAGEMENT

In today's modern health-care arena with the development of new and more sophisticated medication regimes, nursing medication management has become more complex, with increasing responsibility. Medication management is more than medicine administration. Today's modern nurse, in addition to monitoring the effectiveness of treatments, is also expected to advise and educate patients about their individual treatment plans. In the National Health Service (NHS), many medicines are prescribed not only to treat and manage ill health but also to provide a preventative measure. However, it is important to remember that taking medication carries risks and therefore the potential benefits will need to outweigh the associated risks (Healthcare Commission, 2007). To ensure safe and effective medicine management, nurses need to develop understanding of normal and disordered physiology, pharmacology, human behaviour and communication (Nursing and Midwifery Council [NMC], 2007).

Two pieces of legislation regulate medication usage within the United Kingdom. The Medicines Act (1968) is the principle framework for the administration, licensing, sale and supply of medicines in the UK. The Misuse of Drugs Act (1971) controls drugs that have the potential for misuse, regulating the import, export, supply and use of these drugs. Under this act drugs are classified according to their potential to cause harm if abused (classes A, B, C). The Misuse of Drugs Regulations (2001) further classifies into schedules denoting the requirement for import, export, production, supply, possession, prescribing and record-keeping. All health-care professionals involved in medication management must adhere to these acts.

In the clinical setting, whether that be hospital wards, clinics, nursing homes or the patient's own home, nurses repeatedly carry out the administration of medicines. Drug administration has long been and will remain a required competency for entry to the nursing professional register (NMC, 2007). It is also recognised that drug administration is not a routine task but an activity that presents risks not only for the patient but also for the administrator. In recognition of this risk the National Patient Safety Agency (NPSA, 2004) advised that nurses administrating drugs should not be disturbed, allowing total concentration in this task. The NMC (2007, updated 2010) produced standards for medicine management. The aim of this document is to protect the public by producing standards that are broad principles for practice that all registrants need to apply to their own area of practice. As a registrant administrating medication to patients,

- You must be certain of the identity of the patient to whom the medicine is to be administered.
- You must check that the patient is not allergic to the medicine before administering it.
- You must know the therapeutic uses of the medicine to be administered, its normal dosage, side effects, precautions and contraindications.
- You must be aware of the patient's plan of care (care plan or pathway).
- You must check that the prescription or the label on medicine dispensed is clearly written and unambiguous.
- You must check the expiry date (where it exists) of the medicine to be administered.
- You must have considered the dosage, weight where appropriate, method of administration, route and timing.
- You must administer or withhold in the context of the patient's condition (e.g. digoxin is not usually given if the patient's pulse is below 60) and coexisting therapies, for example, physiotherapy.
- You must contact the prescriber or another authorised prescriber without delay if contraindications to the prescribed medicine are discovered, the patient develops a

reaction to the medicine, or assessment of the patient indicates that the medicine is no longer suitable.

- You must make a clear, accurate and immediate record of all medicine administered, intentionally withheld or refused by the patient, ensuring the signature is clear and legible. It is also your responsibility to ensure that a record is made when delegating the task of administering medicine.

In addition:

- If medication is not given, the reason for not doing so must be recorded.
- You may administer with a single signature any prescription-only medicine (POM), general sales list (GSL) or pharmacy (P) medication.

Concerning controlled drugs:

- These should be administered in line with relevant legislation and local standard operating procedures.
- It is recommended that for the administration of controlled drugs a secondary signatory is required within secondary care and similar health-care settings.
- In a patient's home, where a registrant is administering a controlled drug that has already been prescribed and dispensed to that patient, obtaining a secondary signatory should be based on local risk assessment.
- Although normally the second signatory should be another registered health-care professional (e.g. doctor, pharmacist, dentist) or student nurse or midwife, in the interest of patient care, where this is not possible, a second suitable person who has been assessed as competent may sign. It is good practice that the second signatory witnesses the whole administration process. For guidance, the Department of Health (DH) online (https://www.gov.uk/government/organisations/department-of-health) enables searching for safer management of controlled drugs in its guidance on standard operating procedures (see, for example, https://www.gov.uk/government/publications/care-quality-commission-annual-report-2011-on-the-safer-management-of-controlled-drugs).
- In cases of direct patient administration of oral medication from stock in a substance misuse clinic, it must be a registered nurse who administers, with the administration log signed by a second signatory (assessed as competent), who then supervises as the patient receives and consumes the medication.
- You must clearly countersign the signature of the student when supervising a student in the administration of medicines (NMC, 2007).

Also, you must remember the five rights of drug administration:

- Right patient
- Right drug
- Right dose
- Right route
- Right time

Let us now look at the chapter scenario:

Ellen is a 65-year-old retired nurse. She is fit and active, despite taking a non-steroidal anti-inflammatory (NSAID) for arthritis in both knees, which give her occasional pain. Over the last 12 months Ellen has become progressively forgetful and absentminded, often forgetting the names of her friends and misplacing household items. Her husband is becoming increasingly worried about this 'out-of-character' behaviour and has persuaded her to go to her general practitioner (GP) for a checkup.

Is forgetfulness a normal part of the aging process? Can you think of any reasons why Ellen may be forgetful?

Ellen's GP confirms that memory loss is not a normal sign of aging and refers her to the local Memory Clinic. Following a battery of physiological and cognitive assessments, Ellen receives a formal diagnosis of Alzheimer's disease and is commenced on donepezil (Aricept) 5 mg daily.

Ellen remains on Aricept at 5 mg for the recommended 6 weeks and after initial nausea and vomiting, her dose is titrated up to 10 mg daily.

On occasion Ellen forgets to take her medication, often keeping it in her hand for hours at a time before her husband reminds her to swallow it.

Remember, the principles of safe administration of medication apply to all patients, regardless of diagnosis. Supporting the patient to organise his or her daily routine in a way that incorporates the medication regime is vital to living well with dementia (Smith, 2014). Often, assistive technologies can enable people to take their medication safely.

Let us now look at the recommended pharmacological agents for the treatment of Alzheimer's disease.

ANTIDEMENTIA DRUGS

There is no cure for Alzheimer's disease and people who live with dementia may experience a range of often distressing behavioural and psychological symptoms. There are currently three licenced medications available for the treatment of mild to moderate Alzheimer's disease. These therapeutic agents are known as acetylcholinesterase inhibitors (AChEIs) and are donepezil hydrochloride, galantamine hydrobromine, and rivastigmine hydrogen tartrate. Each of the medications may be known in clinical practice by their proprietary or 'trade' name. Do not let this confuse you; the generic name (i.e. the chemical name) will never change.

Each of these medications has been endorsed by the National Institute for Health and Care Excellence (NICE, 2006) and is recognised as having therapeutic value in relieving the *cognitive symptoms* of Alzheimer's disease. The treatment of non-cognitive symptoms is discussed later in the chapter. There are strict prescribing guidelines concerning the initiation of an antidementia drug. In the first instance the person with dementia must have received a formal clinical diagnosis of Alzheimer's disease. This will include examination and assessment of attention and concentration, orientation, short- and long-term memory, praxis, language and executive function.

As part of this assessment, formal cognitive testing should be undertaken using a standardised instrument. The Mini-Mental State Examination (MMSE) has been frequently used for this purpose, but a number of alternatives are now available, such as the 6-Item Cognitive Impairment Test (6CIT), the General Practitioner Assessment of Cognition (GPCOG) and the 7-Minute Screen. Those interpreting the scores of such tests should take full account of other factors known to affect performance, including educational level, skills, prior level of functioning and attainment, language, and any sensory impairments, psychiatric illness or physical/neurological problems (NICE, 2006: 23). Other physiological assessments such as routine blood examinations, urinalysis, or X-ray and structural imaging may also take place depending on clinical presentation.

The three AChEIs are recommended only for people who have a MMSE score of 10–20 points. Only specialists (psychiatrists and neurologists) working in the field of dementia should initiate treatment. Patients' status should be reviewed every 6 months and account taken of their MMSE score as well as global and behavioural functioning. It is imperative that the carer's view of the patient's condition is obtained.

The drug may only be continued whilst the patient's MMSE score remains at or above 10 points or unless the drug is considered to have a positive effect on behaviour and global functioning. It is essential that any side effects are also monitored along with efficacy.

Let us return to the scenario:

Although Ellen's psychiatrist wishes to further titrate the Aricept to the maximum dose of 23 mg, Ellen is unable to tolerate it due to extreme nausea and vomiting, so she remains on 10 mg daily. Ellen's MMSE score remains stable at 20 and her global functioning scores are good. Her husband confirms that she is functioning well.

If a person has been diagnosed with moderate to severe dementia, or as their condition deteriorates, there is a further medication available called memantine (Ebixa) which can be offered. Unlike the three AChEIs (donepezil, galantamine and rivastigmine) discussed previously, memantine is an *N*-methyl-D-aspartate (NMDA) and is licenced for the treatment of moderate to severe Alzheimer's disease or for people who are intolerant to AChEIs. Initiation of the medication and continuation are also subject to strict adherence to NICE guidance (2011).

Remember, it is likely that Ellen will be prescribed memantine as her condition deteriorates.

OTHER PHARMACOLOGICAL INTERVENTIONS

People who live with dementia may also experience depression (Knapskog, Barca, & Knut, 2014). In fact, there is little known about the true prevalence of depression in dementia, and it is often underdiagnosed (its prevalence has been noted to be anywhere between 9% and 68%) (Muliyala & Varghese, 2010). It is recommended that people with dementia and a comorbid depressive disorder be offered antidepressant medication (NICE, 2006). However, pharmacological treatment should only be initiated by staff with specialist training and should follow the NICE Clinical Guidance *Depression in Adults: The Treatment and Management of Depression in Adults* (NICE, 2009a). Monitoring of side effects and age-appropriate dosage must also be considered. Psychological therapies can also be an effective intervention.

Let us revisit the scenario:

Despite living well with dementia, Ellen has been experiencing intermittent episodes of low mood. Because of this her GP prescribes her a selective serotonin reuptake inhibitor (SSRI), citalopram 20 mg. Furthermore, Ellen reports that her 'knees are getting worse', for which she takes aspirin when required.

SSRIs are associated with an increased risk of bleeding, especially in older people or in people taking other drugs that are associated with serious gastrointestinal toxicity (BNF.org, 2015). Can you identify any medication that Ellen is taking that would cause concern? Remember that Ellen has arthritis and takes an NSAID along with aspirin when required.

Everyone experiences pain throughout life, which can be physical pain such as toothache, backache, headache or emotional pain such as bereavement. Often the experience of pain is what prompts patients to seek help. In the past pain was viewed as a necessity of an illness that needed to be endured by the patient. Our understanding of pain has deepened and we are now aware that pain is what patients fear most, and if present can hinder the healing process. Understanding what can cause pain and what can be done about pain enables us to provide high standards of care.

Pain differs in many ways and is dependent on the individual experience which may be influenced by factors such as culture, values, fear, anxiety, prognosis and diagnosis. It is important that we listen to our patients and how they describe their pain. A patient may describe the pain as boring, nagging, stabbing, shooting, crushing or aching. To assess pain we may wish to record the intensity or strength of pain by using pain scales, which can be in the form of a visual analogue scale using a 10-cm line ranging from no pain to worst possible pain, a numerical pain intensity scale from 1 to 10 or face diagrams that show feelings from a grimace to a smiley face.

When assessing pain we need to ascertain the circumstances associated with pain onset: primary site of pain, any radiation to other parts of the body, character of the pain (boring, nagging, stabbing, shooting, crushing or aching), intensity, precipitating and relieving factors, timing, and the effect of the pain on the patient (activities, sleep). We also need to know what the patient has done about the pain and whether the patient has taken any medication or used any nonpharmacological treatments (e.g. heat/cold packs, etc.).

People who live with dementia—particularly those who live in nursing or residential homes—are at risk of underrecognition and undertreatment of pain (Newton et al., 2014). Constipation, urinary tract infections and toothache are some things that cause great discomfort and distress. And while it can be difficult to assess pain when a person living with dementia may not be able to communicate distress using conventional methods, it is important to remember that the person's experience of pain is not altered due to dementia. The therapeutic approach and the ability to detect often subtle behavioural changes are crucial to a pain assessment for a person with dementia. Features such as agitation, fidgeting, facial grimacing, wailing and signs of distress on physical examination are observable signs of pain. If a carer's input can be supplied then every effort should be made to seek it. A thorough assessment and the prescribing of painkillers can bring about great relief for people who live with dementia and improve their quality of life.

Let us look again at the scenario:

Ellen's husband contacts the memory service as he is concerned that Ellen is experiencing severe pain in her knees and consequently taking more than the recommended dose of aspirin.

The mental health practitioner and community pharmacist visit Ellen at home and recommend that Ellen stop taking aspirin and instead take paracetamol on prescription.

A referral to the rheumatology clinic is initiated at this time. The mental health practitioner also offers some lifestyle advice around exercise and diet.

Drugs used to control pain range from mild, over-the-counter preparations to general anaesthetics.

The World Health Organisation (WHO, 1986) proposed a simple, reliable and effective way of pain management called the 'analgesic ladder'.

Step 1: Mild pain to be managed with nonopioid analgesics, antipyretics and nonsteroidal NSAIDs.

Step 2: Moderate pain and those who are not pain free on step 1 to be managed with weak opioid analgesia with additional nonopioid drugs.

Step 3: Severe pain or those who are not pain free on step 2 to be managed on strong opioid.

Nonopioid analgesics are normally aspirin, ibuprofen or paracetamol. Paracetamol is generally preferred as it does not have as many side effects as aspirin or ibruprofen. Aspirin (derived from willow bark) has a long history but it was not until the end of the nineteenth century that it was first patented. Aspirin has good analgesic, anti-inflammatory, antipyretic and antiplatelet properties. It is thought to act by blocking the cyclooxygenase pathway; however by doing so it may produce side effects involving the digestive tract and kidneys. Ibuprofen also works by blocking the cyclooxygenase pathway so it has similar effect for mild to moderate pain. Paracetamol (discovered over 100 years ago) is used to relieve pain and fever. It does not appear to have any anti-inflammatory or antiplatelet effect and therefore has much fewer side effects than aspirin or ibuprofen. It is thought that its mechanism of action is via cyclooxygenase 3 inhibition. It is important to be aware that paracetamol is dangerous when taken in excess.

Opioid analgesics are given for moderate to severe pain when nonopioid analgesics are ineffective. They are derived from the opium poppy and have been used for centuries. All centrally acting opioid analgesics work by stimulating receptors within the central nervous system. These receptors react to naturally occurring compounds within our body that can reduce our response to painful stimuli. However due to the range of receptors involved, opioid analgesics, while reducing pain, can also affect mood by producing euphoria, respiratory depression, cough reflex depression, nausea, vomiting and pupillary constriction.

As discussed earlier, people who live with dementia can experience a range of behavioural and psychological symptoms, often referred to as BPSD (behavioural and psychological symptoms in dementia). Such symptoms can include agitation, aggression, wandering and shouting and can significantly complicate care (DH, 2009).

BPSD are common, and are distressing for both patients and carers. They are frequently the reason for admission to nursing home care. Treating BPSD is not easy. Historically, people who experienced BPSD were treated with antipsychotic medications. The Banerjee report *The Use of Antipsychotic Medication for People Who Live with Dementia: A Time for Action* (DH, 2009) argued that antipsychotic medications were overused, inappropriately used, have minimal effect on BPSD and actually pose more harm than benefit to patients. The risks of prescribing antipsychotic medication to people who live with dementia are now well attested in the literature.

In light of this, Banerjee (DH, 2009) proposed that only specialists in the field of dementia be involved in the decisions concerning initiation, review and cessation of antipsychotic medication. Furthermore, the Banerjee report called for more psychosocial interventions, including educating and increasing skills of carers and better use of the Improving Access to Psychological Therapies (IAPT) services for people who live with dementia.

For now, Ellen is not exhibiting any BPSD. Given the recommendations of the Banerjee report, can you think about some interventions that might be useful as Ellen's condition worsens?

Ellen and her husband have started to visit a 'dementia café' at their local community centre. Here, they are involved in a range of psychosocial activities ranging from reminiscence and art therapy to aromatherapy and hand massage. Her husband has noticed that Ellen's mood seems to be improving, and they both enjoy the social engagement.

PRESCRIBING

Traditionally, prescribing has been a medically dominated activity; however since the early 1990s this crucial health-care activity has been extended to other health professionals. The extension of prescribing rights has been driven by the need to modernise the NHS, ensuring capacity to deliver accessible and high-quality care to patients. Modernisation has been achieved by expanding the roles of existing health-care professionals whilst maintaining patient safety. Appropriately qualified nurses, pharmacists and allied health professionals can now prescribe medication within their clinical competence and as permitted within legislative framework. Mental health nurse prescribing is seen as an exciting development and has the potential to enhance service provision (Ross & Kettles, 2012).

Suitably qualified mental health nurses first gained access to prescribing rights across England in April 2003. Initially they were only able to act as extended and supplementary prescribers, prescribing through a patient-specific clinical management plan formulated collaboratively with a doctor and patient, and based on a diagnosis established by a doctor. In 2006, the British National Formulary (BNF) was opened up to appropriately qualified nurses and pharmacists. Within their area of competence, independent prescribers can diagnose and prescribe any licensed medicines and some controlled drugs without supervision from a doctor.

Evidence suggests that non-medical prescribing benefits patients through improvements in service delivery and better use of staff skills (Jones & Edwards, 2011). However as Nutall (2013) observes, to achieve this the competence of the prescriber is fundamental. The National Prescribing Centre (NPC, 2012) stresses the necessity for practitioners to prescribe only within their boundaries of competence—a view supported by professional bodies including the NMC (2015) and the General Pharmaceutical Council (GPhC, 2012). The NPC provides a framework which includes key principles to guide prescribing practice (NPC, 1999), a validated and versatile tool to assist all prescribers in achieving and maintaining competence. The 'Standards of Proficiency for Nurse and Midwife Prescribers' (NMC, 2006) sets standards to assist prescribers to ensure their competence and safety.

Nurses in the UK are required to be qualified as nurses for at least 3 years and educated to degree level before starting the prescribing course. Courses are held at higher educational institutes over 3–6 months and consist of 26 days theory plus additional self-directed study. A portfolio demonstrating knowledge and competence in the prescriber's specialist area must be completed along with a pharmacology and numeracy exam.

It is easy to become confused by the types of non-medical prescribing in existence.

The medicinal products: Prescription by Nurses Act (1992) is legislation within the Medicines Act that permitted nurses to prescribe for the first time. This act allowed district nurses and health visitors who had successfully completed a recommended programme to become registered with the NMC as prescribers. These prescribers could prescribe from the Nurse Prescribers Formulary.

V100: This is community practitioner prescribing that allows nurse practitioners who have completed the appropriate qualifications that allow access to prescribe from that specific formulary only.

V150: Noncommunity nurse practitioners who are appropriately qualified and recorded on the NMC register are allowed to access the community practitioner formulary only.

V300: This is in regard to independent and supplementary prescribers—nurses who have appropriate qualifications and record on the NMC register with access to prescribe any medicine for any medical condition. Nurse independent prescribers are able to prescribe, administer, and give directions for the administration of Schedule 2, 3, 4, and 5 controlled drugs. This extends to diamorphine, dipipanone, or cocaine for treating disease or injury, but not for treating addiction (British National Formulary [BNF], 68).

Supplementary prescribing: This is 'a voluntary partnership between an independent prescriber (doctor or dentist) and a supplementary prescriber (nurse, pharmacist or Allied Health Professional) to implement an agreed patient specific clinical management plan with the patient's agreement' (DH, 2003).

The same training programme qualifies nurses for both supplementary prescribers and independent non-medical prescribers, with a generic preparation common to all nursing specialties. Nurses are required to ensure that their prescribing practice remains within their area of competence and the limits of their knowledge (DH, 2007).

Latter et al. (2011) concluded that while service users do not have a particular preference for nurse or doctor prescribers, certain attributes within prescribing consultations are particularly valued, including the ability to listen to service users' views and provide good information. Earle et al. (2011) reported that although service users were generally positive about nurse prescribing, improvement could be made with regards to sharing information about medications.

The potential of non-medical prescribing in mental health is increasingly being recognized, with a significant increase in the number of nurses undertaking prescribing training. As numbers increase, so does the need to ensure that appropriate governance and safeguards are in place. Methods by which independent prescribers can be supported in practice need to be strengthened, while recognizing the valuable role of nurse prescribers in promoting adherence among those with severe and enduring mental illness (Dobel-Ober, Brimblecombe, & Bradley, 2013).

NICE guidelines (2009b) advise that when deciding on treatment options, adherence and possible side effects should be taken into consideration. It is important that practitioners acknowledge that the decision to prescribe treatment must take into account the patient's views and preferences, and that the patient must be involved in the treatment decision. This style of consultation is known as concordance or shared decision-making (Petty, 2012).

CHAPTER SUMMARY

The principles of medication management are applicable to all patient groups; however, this chapter discussed best practice in relation to people living with dementia.

The pharmacological interventions for both the cognitive and non-cognitive symptoms of dementia have been examined along with the supporting national guidance.

The subject of pain and the according subtleties when assessing and treating someone with dementia have been explored.

Because national guidance, legislation and best practice are subject to change as the evidence base increases and expands, it is vital to keep up to date with the change in our ever-changing health-care world.

REFLECTION ON LEARNING

1. Can you name the two pieces of legislation which regulate medication usage within the United Kingdom?
2. Is the safe administration of medication a competency for entry to the professional register?
3. Describe what is meant by the 'Five Rs' of drug administration.
4. Can you name the three AChEIs?
5. According to NICE (2011), at what point on the MMSE should an antidementia drug be discontinued?
6. How common is depression amongst people living with dementia?
7. Why is it not advised to prescribe antipsychotic medication to people who live with dementia and experience BPSD?
8. How many steps are in the WHO (1986) analgesia ladder?
9. What are the possible side effects of opioid analgesics?
10. Who can legally prescribe medication in the United Kingdom?

REFERENCES

British National Formulary (BNF) (67). http://www.bnf.org/

BNF.org. 2015. *British National Formulary* (68). http://www.bnf.org/bnf/index.htm.

Department of Health. 2003. *Supplementary Prescribing by Nurses and Pharmacists within the NHS in England: A Guide for Implementation*. London: Department of Health.

Department of Health. 2007. Clinical Management Plans (CMPs). http://www .dh.gov.uk/en/healthcare/medicinespharmacyandindustry/prescriptions/ thenonmedicalprescribingprogramme/supplementaryprescribing/dh-4123030.

Department of Health. 2009. *The Use of Antipsychotic Medication for People with Dementia: Time for Action*. A report for the Minister of State for Care Services by Professor Sube Banerjee. London: Department of Health.

Dobel-Ober, D., Brimblecombe, N., & Bradley, E. 2013. An evaluation of team and individual formularies to support independent prescribing in mental health care. *Journal of Psychiatric and Mental Health Nursing*, 20: 35–40.

Earle, E.A., Taylor, J., Peet, M., & Grant, G. 2011. Nurse prescribing in specialist mental health (Part 1): The views and experiences of practicing and non-practicing nurse prescribers and service users. *Journal of Psychiatric and Mental Health Nursing*, 18: 189–197.

General Pharmaceutical Council. 2012. *Standards of Conduct, Ethics and Performance*. London: General Pharmaceutical Council.

Healthcare Commission. 2007. *The Best Medicine: The Management of Medicines in Acute and Specialist Trusts*. London: Commission for Healthcare Audit and Inspection.

Jones, K., & Edwards, M. 2011. Nurse prescribing roles in acute care: an evaluative case study. *Journal of Advanced Nursing*, 67: 117–126.

Knapskog, A., Barca, M.J., & Knut, E. 2014. Prevalence of depression amongst memory clinic patients as measured by the Cornell Scale of Depression in Dementia. *Aging and Mental Health*, 18(5): 579–587.

Latter, S., Blenkinsopp, A., Smith, A., Smith, A., Chapman, S., Tinelli, M., Gerard, K., Little, Paul, Celino, N., Granby, T., et al. 2011. *Evaluation of Nurse and Pharmacist Independent Prescribing*. London: Department of Health.

Medicines Act 1968. London: the Stationary Office. http://www.legislation.gov.uk/ukpga/1968/67

Medicinal Products: Prescription by Nurses etc. Act 1992. http://www.legislation.gov.uk/ukpga/1992/28/contents

Misuse of Drugs Act 1971. London: the Stationary Office. http://www.legislation.gov.uk/ukpga/1971/38/contents

Misuse of Drugs Regulation 2001. London: the Stationary Office. http://www.legislation.gov.uk/uksi/2001/3998/contents/made

Muliyala, K., & Varghese, M. 2010. The complex relationship between depression and dementia. *Annals of Indian Academy of Neurology*, 13(6): 69–73.

National Institute for Health and Clinical Excellence. 2006. *Dementia: Supporting People with Dementia and Their Carers in Health and Social Care*. London: NICE.

National Institute for Health and Clinical Excellence. 2009a. *Depression in Adults. The Treatment and Management of Depression in Adults*. NICE Clinical Guideline 90. London: NICE.

National Institute for Health and Clinical Excellence. 2009b. *Depression: Treatment and Management of Depression in Adults with a Chronic Physical Health Problem*. London: NICE.

National Institute for Health and Clinical Excellence. 2011. *Donepezil, Galantamine, Rivastigmine and Memantine for the Treatment of Alzheimer's Disease*. NICE Technological Appraisal Guidance 217. London: NICE.

National Patient Safety Agency. 2004. Seven Steps to Patient Safety: An Overview Guide for NHS Staff. http://www.npsa.nhs.co.uk/patientsafety/improvingpatientsafety/7steps/.

National Prescribing Centre. 1999. Signposts for prescribing nurses: General principles of good prescribing. *Nurse Bulletin*, 1(1): 1–4.

National Prescribing Centre. 2012. A Single Competency Framework for All Prescribers. http://www.npc.co,uk/improving safety/improving quality/resoures/single compframework.pdf.

Newton, P., Reeves, R., West, E., & Schofield, P. 2014. Patient centred assessment and management of pain for older adults with dementia in care home and acute settings. *Reviews in Clinical Gerontology*, 24: 139–144.

Nursing and Midwifery Council. 2006. *Standards of Proficiency for Nurse and Midwife Prescribers*.

Nursing and Midwifery Council. 2007. Standards for Medicines Management. http://www.nmc-uk.org.

Nursing and Midwifery Council. 2010. *Standards for Pre-registration Nursing Education*. London: Nursing and Midwifery Council.

Nursing and Midwifery Council. 2015. *The Code: Professional Standards of Practice and Behaviour for Nurses and Midwives*. London: Nursing and Midwifery Council.

Nutall, D. 2013. Self-assessing competence in non-medical prescribing. *Nurse Prescribing*, 8: 66–69.

Petty, D.R. 2012. Ten tips for safer prescribing by non-medical prescribers. *Nurse Prescribing*, 10: 251–256.

Prescription by Nurses Act. 1992. London: the Stationary Office.

Ross, J.D., & Kettles, A. 2012. Mental health nurse independent prescribing: What are nurse prescribers' views of the barriers to implementation? *Journal of Psychiatric and Mental Health Nursing*, 19: 916–932.

Smith, G. 2014. *Mental Health Nursing at a Glance*. Chichester, UK: Wiley Blackwell.

World Health Organization. 1987. *Cancer Pain Relief*. Geneva, Switzerland: World Health Organization.

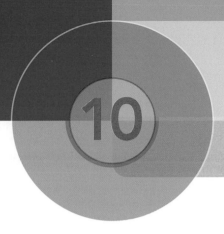

Psychological interventions in dementia

DEBORAH KNOTT AND DENISE PARKER

AIM

- To explore psychological interventions in dementia

OBJECTIVES

- To be familiar with a range of effective communication skills
- To understand the importance of building a sustainable therapeutic relationship
- To consider the application of a number of psychological interventions: cognitive-focused approaches, behavioural therapy interventions, and interventions for comorbid conditions such as depression and anxiety

OVERVIEW

For the purposes of this chapter a psychological intervention is broadly understood as a health and social care intervention (Smith, 2012) 'which is underpinned by psychological methods and theory with the intention of improving biopsychosocial functioning, it is usually delivered through therapeutically structured relationship' (p. 2). For psychological interventions to be successful, these must be delivered, using effective communication, within a therapeutic relationship. Good communication alone is not sufficient to deliver a range of effective interventions; rather, a therapeutic relationship and, within it, the interpersonal skills that build this relationship are the foundation with which effective interventions are built (O'Carroll & Park, 2007; Knott, 2012). Any interventions delivered should be clinically effective and evidence based, and they should also consider the values that are inherent within the therapeutic relationship (Smith, 2012).

In dementia care, the evidence base on the use of psychological interventions is continually strengthening. There are still gaps, especially in relation to psychological interventions for people with early dementia (Moniz-Cook & Manthorpe, 2009; Parker, 2012). The gaps in this area stem from studies focusing on people with dementia who have complex symptoms and the challenges that carers, formal and informal, have in meeting those challenges (Parker, 2012). There is a need to plug this gap, particularly where there is a drive throughout the UK to increase early diagnosis rates (DH, 2009; DHSSPS, 2011; Welsh Assembly Government, 2011; Scottish Government, 2013). Upon receiving an early diagnosis a person with dementia and their carer(s) require a service that is fit for purpose and includes the ability to access psychological interventions that are underpinned by a robust evidence base (Alzheimer's Society, 2014).

Psychological interventions in dementia care are heavily influenced by Tom Kitwood's work on personhood. Kitwood's work tends to be understood by health and social care practitioners as person-centred care (Parker, 2012; Mast, 2014). Being person-centred, according to Mast (2014), acknowledges that people with dementia should be given 'respect, honour, and value' (p. 291). Sometimes the practitioner, especially when busy, may focus on symptom control rather than the person (Kitwood, 1997; Parker, 2012). On this basis it is vital when building therapeutic relationships with those with dementia to keep in mind the concept of personhood in all interactions and whatever the context (Kitwood, 1997; Parker, 2012; Mast, 2014).

Agnes is a 78-year-old woman who has had a diagnosis of Alzheimer's disease for almost 2 years. She lives alone in her own home supported by her two daughters and two grandchildren, who have been supportive and are vocal regarding Agnes's needs. They are struggling with Agnes's growing confusion. There has been an initial meeting with Agnes and her family at which the family was clear in what they thought Agnes needed to stay in her own home. Agnes appeared confused throughout this meeting and was unable to answer any but the most basic questions.

Agnes wears a hearing aid which she often forgets to turn on or forgets to wear altogether. A key worker is assigned and a followup visit is due to assess Agnes's level of functioning with a view to working with her and her family to manage her symptoms.

EFFECTIVE COMMUNICATION

Communication should be a two-way process: The health and social care practitioner works in partnership with people living with dementia, a 'doing with' rather than a 'doing to' approach (Knott, 2012). To create a sustainable therapeutic relationship which is collaborative and underpinned by effective communication, the practitioner has to be self-aware (Knott, 2012; Smith, 2014). Understanding the self is a key component of being an effective communicator. Most health and social care preregistration programmes will provide the opportunity for practitioners to work on the development of self as an effective communicator, however this is not a journey that stops at the point of registration. It is an ongoing journey—a lifelong learning journey (Nursing and Midwifery Council, 2010; Knott, 2012; Smith, 2014).

The majority of communication is nonverbal, or what is called body language. This type of communication is most powerful when a person does not comprehend the words that are being spoken or cannot convey personal wants and wishes through language (Knott, 2012; Foley & Gentile, 2010). This is particularly true when working in the dementia care setting where a person with dementia may lose the ability to communicate verbally, leaving the carer to pick up on nonverbal cues and body language (Allan & Killick, 2014). There are many challenges when communicating with those who experience dementia, which appear to be consistent across the age barrier or the environmental setting. Persons with dementia experience vagueness; they forget words so, for example, instead of using the word *spade* they may say 'that thing you dig a hole with'. These are called circumlocutions, and the caregiver will become used to these as the relationship develops and interpretation becomes easier. In addition, disrupted coherence and cohesion may be displayed by which the person is extremely verbal yet makes little sense, using incomplete sentences and incorrect words (Bourgeois & Hickey, 2009). The more general characteristics of dementia that also influence communication include difficulties with memory and impaired cognitive and executive abilities (WHO, 2012). Add to this issues with distorted perception (e.g. loss of hearing or impaired vision) that often comes with the aging process and effective communication becomes difficult.

Environmentally, should the person be living with dementia in a care home, there is often increased passivity and lack of expectation caused by the environment, such as high sound levels, lack of privacy, and less-than-ideal seating arrangements (Van Zadelhoff et al., 2011). The seating arrangements may preclude conversation, with seats being placed too far apart to allow decent conversation.

To combat these difficulties, the general principles of good communication should be applied, particularly maintaining eye contact and paying close attention to nonverbal cues and body language (Knott, 2012). Returning to the chapter scenario:

On the first visit the key worker is accompanied by a student who observes the key worker's interactions. After the visit the student is asked to reflect on their observations. The student noticed that the key worker utilised a one-to-one approach, sitting close to Agnes, maintaining eye contact and speaking clearly and deliberately, but not in what could be interpreted as a patronising manner. When testing Agnes's functioning, the key worker used instructions that were broken down into simple phrases and only gave one instruction at a time, therefore limiting choices and options. Open-ended questions were avoided—the key worker explained that this could be tricky as it is against usual principles of good communication. The topics discussed were limited and Agnes was encouraged to talk about herself and her experiences, with the key worker using prompts and cues to prevent Agnes getting 'lost' in the conversation.

THE THERAPEUTIC RELATIONSHIP

Extensive behavioural and social evidence supports the growing need for a person-centred approach for those living with dementia. The nature of this approach within a health and social care context means that it needs to be delivered within a therapeutic relationship (Kitwood 1997; Mast, 2014; Parker, 2012; Allan & Killick, 2014). People with dementia respond well to personal contact so in a sense it is the contact and not the activity that builds the relationship. Any such contact needs to be within a routine as much as possible and include family members and carers to develop a consistent approach (Allan & Killick, 2014). Within this approach, treatments will work best in specific, time-limited situations tailored to individuals' requirements and delivered within a trusting, therapeutic alliance (Allan & Killick, 2014).

A therapeutic relationship is a purposeful and positive relationship by which the practitioner assists the service user in the user's journey to recovery (Rigby & Alexander, 2008). However recovery is a concept not usually associated with dementia care. In this instance *recovery* is taken to mean enabling the service user to live the best life possible whilst receiving care from dementia services (Parker, 2012; Smith, 2014). Therapeutic relationships should be both evidence based and values based. They should deliver positive therapeutic outcomes, and the practitioner should be committed to working in partnership with people living with dementia and other practitioners (Smith, 2012).

At times it can be difficult for the practitioner to reconstruct a person's own experience of mental distress, particularly if the person with dementia finds it difficult to express this distress (Allan & Killick, 2014). This can happen, for example, when a conversation only captures the information the practitioner needs (e.g. assessment information) but does not capture the service user's entire story (Smith, 2012). Having different viewpoints can create conflict within the relationship unless the mental health nurse takes a collaborative approach. In addition, the therapeutic relationship within dementia care has a 'risk element' which may shape the relationship in some way. The impact is that even though the therapeutic relationship is intended to be collaborative and person centred, this intention can be dependent on the level of risk and the caregiver's need to keep the person with dementia safe (Smith, 2012). Even so, the practitioner should always look to build therapeutic relationships that are based on true partnership work and at the same time value both the service user and the user's experiences, a person-centred philosophy (Parker, 2012; Mast, 2014).

To be truly collaborative the practitioner has to be self-aware, particularly when working with those with dementia. It is difficult for us to understand how the person may be feeling, having not experienced this ourselves. The practitioner has to be aware of the impact their self has on others; they need to be aware of their own thoughts and feelings, and they also need to be able to use this knowledge in a positive way when working with people with dementia (Allan & Killick, 2014). It is essential within the therapeutic relationship that the practitioner is empathic, meaning that the practitioner has to be able to identify with the service user's experiences throughout (Knott, 2012) by 'conveying genuine interest, acceptance and caring' (p. 31). We now return to Agnes:

The key worker has visited Agnes on four occasions in her home and Agnes is beginning to accept the key worker as someone who she sees regularly, although she is unable to remember the key worker's name or the purpose of the visits and remains initially suspicious. To build the therapeutic relationship and then initially engage with Agnes during visits the key worker talks with Agnes about her interests, such as watching TV 'soaps'; this information was identified during the assessment process.

COGNITIVE-FOCUSED INTERVENTIONS

By developing effective communication skills the practitioner will have a good foundation on which to develop a range of psychological interventions intended to meet the needs of those living with dementia (Knott, 2012). This further development should include psychological interventions that are designed to support a person's cognitive abilities.

Managing life with increasing cognitive impairment is at the centre of adapting to living with dementia. Damage to cognitive functions often starts with memory impairment, and progressively widens to other cognitive functions and worsens. (Oyebode & Clare, 2014: 189)

According to Oyebode and Clare (2014), cognitive-focused interventions can be divided into three main approaches:

1. Cognitive training
2. Cognitive stimulation
3. Cognitive rehabilitation

Cognitive training is an approach that involves the person with dementia being guided to practice and complete a set of cognitive tasks which involve cognitive functions such as memory, attention, and problem solving (Parker, 2012; Oyebode & Clare, 2014). Cognitive training is an intense approach. Sessions can be 30 to 60 minutes in duration, with a frequency of three to seven times weekly. These sessions can be delivered by formal and informal carers using paper and pencil or computer programmes and in a variety of settings (Parker, 2012; Oyebode & Clare, 2014). Flexibility is an important part of this approach, however this makes it more difficult to measure effectiveness (Oyebode & Clare, 2014).

Cognitive stimulation incorporates reality orientation activities (focusing on time, place, and person) and reminiscence activities, using past memories to provoke thinking (cognition), conversation, and social interaction (Oyebode & Clare, 2014; Parker, 2012). In terms of clinical guidelines, this approach is recommended. There is also significant evidence that it is an effective approach for people with mild to moderate dementia when delivered at least once a week (NCCMH, 2007/2011; Oyebode & Clare, 2014; Parker, 2012).

Cognitive rehabilitation is a psychological intervention which is underpinned by person-centred philosophy. It is usually delivered on an individual basis rather than as a group intervention (Parker, 2012). Interventions are tailor-made and goal focused; the person with dementia will be supported to work on an everyday task such as taking medication safely. The person will practice the task and the memories associated with the task, name of the medication and time they need to take the medication. Prompting is used which includes the use of memory-enabling aids (Oyebode & Clare, 2014). There is promising evidence through small-scale studies and a single randomized controlled trial that this approach has potential (Oyebode & Clare, 2014). Let us return to the chapter scenario:

The key worker has started to work with Agnes and her family to increase Agnes's social interaction and stimulate her memory. One strategy the family has adopted is to produce a memory box for Agnes which is filled with photographs of important events or people, such as her wedding day and her children. There are a number of photographs of the seaside, which is one of Agnes's favourite places. The key worker supports Agnes and her family to plan a day trip.

BEHAVIOUR-FOCUSED INTERVENTIONS

There is little research evidence that concentrates on behavioural therapy as a stand-alone model of treatment for dementia, however it is often the behaviour of persons living with dementia that is the cause of most distress to the persons and their carers (Parker, 2012). The behaviours being displayed, including memory loss, wandering and anxiety, and incontinence provide increasing challenges to all those involved with dementia, whether early in the experience and struggling with fear and depression or later in the illness when family members are no longer recognised and the person becomes incontinent (Parker, 2012).

Behaviour therapy in its purest form looks at specific, learned behaviours and how the environment impacts on those behaviours. Its aim is to modify these behaviours, often through a reward or 'token economy' system in which the subject is rewarded for changing his or her problematic behaviour. This type of therapy can be seen in many areas within the field of psychology (star charts for rewarding good behaviour in children, e.g.). It is a matter of ethical consideration as to whether this type of modification of behaviour would be suitable or effective for those living with dementia. It could be argued that rewarding good behaviour is archaic and as memory is a problem, the service user would be unable to effectively engage in pure behaviour therapy (Cohen-Mansfield, 2014). Cohen-Mansfield (2014) argue that what is viewed as challenging behaviour in dementia is in reality an expression of an unmet need. These needs include (Cohen-Mansfield, 2014):

- Being in physical pain and discomfort
- Being too hot or cold
- Wanting social contact and stimulation
- Experiencing mental distress

When confronted by what is routinely called 'challenging behaviour' a simple but effective approach is to consider whether all the person's needs are being met, if the person is in pain, if the person feels lonely, whether the building is too hot, or if the person is seeing things that are not there. Using memory aids including computer programmes that include pictures of the environment and surroundings, narratives of life stories, and family photographs can improve orientation to a person's surroundings and the important people in the person's life (Oyebode & Clare, 2014). This in turn can have a positive impact on the ability of a person living with dementia to identify names and faces and areas with which they are familiar, which can assist in reducing stress and feelings of isolation, increase cognitive functioning and social interaction and be extremely useful in building relationships with both formal and informal carers (Oyebode & Clare, 2014; Cohen-Mansfield, 2014). Returning to Agnes:

Agnes's family is concerned that at times Agnes appears agitated and on occasion wanders at night. Agnes's key worker reassures the family that there are many simple and practical techniques that can have a positive impact on Agnes's behaviour. These include the following:

- Keeping Agnes active during the day and promoting a restful environment at night
- Providing daily reminders of date, time and place through calendars, newspapers and verbal reminders
- Placing notices on doors regarding locking the door or not leaving the house after dark
- Placing notices on the doors within the living environment (e.g. to indicate bathroom and toilet)
- Providing family photographs with the family members labelled using Post-it® notes

---

INTERVENTIONS FOR DEPRESSION AND ANXIETY

Experiencing anxiety and depression is common in people with dementia and their carers. Psychological interventions have been suggested as a potential treatment for the symptoms (Parker, 2012; Zarit & Zarit, 2014; Paukert et al., 2010; Orgeta et al., 2014). This suggestion has to be set against the view that suggests that people with dementia have limited opportunities for psychological treatments aimed at improving their well-being overall, as treatment tends to focus on memory functioning (Paukert et al., 2010). There is evidence that psychological interventions added to usual care can reduce symptoms of depression and anxiety for people with dementia and therefore have the potential to improve overall patient well-being (Hogan et al., 2008).

Depression and dementia commonly coexist and are associated with higher rates of behavioural and functional problems. In addition caregivers of these individuals report higher levels of physical and mental distress. Effective treatment, therefore, has the potential to help both the older adult and their caregiver (Parker, 2012; Zarit & Zarit, 2014; Paukert et al., 2010). A psychosocial approach should examine all aspects of depression and anxiety and how they impact on the person's quality of life, outside the dementia diagnosis (Woods, 2012; Parker, 2012). The practicality of assisting the person with dementia in managing real feelings of depression and anxiety is problematic. Many of the techniques would be difficult for the person with a cognitive impairment to grasp, remember and practice. However with the guidance and assistance of carers there are several techniques that have proved useful (Parker, 2012; Woods, 2012; Paukert et al., 2010; Hogan et al., 2008).

A problem solving approach, using modified cognitive-behavioural methods with the therapy delivered at a slower pace, using repetition to ensure understanding, works well. The collaboration between the caregiver, the person with dementia and the therapist provides support and encouragement while cementing the therapeutic relationship. Communication is key, and pictures, drawings and written instructions are used as visual aids to supplement verbal cues (Oyebode & Clare, 2014; Paukert et al., 2010; Hogan et al., 2008). The implementation of a deep breathing technique is relatively simple to perform and is proven to work for anxiety symptoms. This can be developed into more in-depth muscle relaxation techniques or guided discovery types of anxiety management sessions depending on the cognitive ability of the person. All these interventions can be carried out in the absence of the therapist, using the carer or audio visual aids (Woods, 2012; Paukert et al., 2010; Hogan et al., 2008).

It is important to recognise that any type of psychological intervention needs to be individualised and set to the correct pace. Sessions need to be shortened, with frequent breaks, and should not be used in isolation but form part of a plan of individualised care delivery (Mast, 2014; Parker, 2012).

Cognitive behavioural strategies can provide both the emotional support and the skills needed for the newly diagnosed person to manage and come to terms with their diagnosis and should be implemented in collaboration with all caregivers involved (Parker, 2012). Let us return to Agnes:

Agnes is becoming increasingly wary of answering her door. She needs a great deal of persuasion to leave her home, even with her daughters, and she is constantly worrying about her finances. She has displayed periods of crying but is unable to give a reason for her upset. Her appetite has reduced and she is getting out of bed later in the mornings.

Agnes is displaying symptoms of anxiety. The key worker produces a care plan with Agnes and her family that focuses on addressing these issues through guided relaxation and deep breathing.

CHAPTER SUMMARY

A psychological intervention is a health and social care intervention which is underpinned by psychological methods and theory with the intention of improving biopsychosocial functioning. It is usually delivered through a therapeutically structured relationship. For psychological interventions to be successful, it is vital that these are delivered using effective communication and within a therapeutic relationship.

Communication is a two-way process with the health and social care practitioner working in partnership with people living with dementia using a doing with rather than a doing to approach. The medium for this approach is the therapeutic relationship, which is a purposeful and positive relationship that enables a person with dementia to live the best life possible. Possessing effective communication skills provides the practitioner with a good foundation on which to develop a range of psychological interventions.

Psychological interventions that are cognitively focused are designed to support a person's cognitive abilities. There are three main approaches: cognitive training, cognitive stimulation, and cognitive rehabilitation.

Behaviour-focused interventions should be based on the premise that challenging behaviour in dementia is in reality an expression of an unmet need. When confronted by what is routinely called 'challenging behaviour', a simple but effective approach is to consider whether all of the person's needs are being met.

Experiencing anxiety and depression is common in people living with dementia; on this basis, psychological interventions have been suggested as a potential treatment for these symptoms. This has to be set against the view that suggests that people with dementia have limited opportunities for psychological treatments. However, there is evidence that psychological interventions can reduce symptoms of depression and anxiety for people with dementia.

REFLECTION ON LEARNING

1. What are psychological interventions? How are they used within a dementia context?
2. Who is Tom Kitwood?
3. What type of process should communication be?
4. How does the environment impact on communication?
5. Define recovery within a dementia context.
6. Why is empathy so important?
7. What is the relationship between cognitive stimulation, reality orientation, and reminiscence?
8. Identify an unmet need.
9. What other mental health conditions are commonly associated with dementia?
10. Describe a modified cognitive behavioural approach.

REFERENCES

Allan, K., & Killick, J. 2014. Communication and relationships: An inclusive social world. In *Excellence in Dementia Care: Research into Practice*, 2nd edition, edited by Downs, M., & Bowers, B., 240–255. Maidenhead, UK: Open University Press.

Alzheimer's Society. 2014. *Dementia 2014: Opportunity for Change*. London: Alzheimer's Society.

Bourgeois, M.S., & Hickey, E.M. 2009. *Dementia: From Diagnosis to Management—A Functional Approach*. New York: Taylor & Francis Group.

Cohen-Mansfield, J. 2014. Understanding behaviour. In *Excellence in Dementia Care*, 2nd edition, edited by Downs, M., & Bowers, B., 220–239. Maidenhead, UK: Open University Press.

Department of Health. 2009. *Living Well with Dementia: A National Dementia Strategy*. London: Department of Health.

Department of Health, Social Services and Public Safety. 2011. *Improving Dementia Services in Northern Ireland: A Regional Strategy*. Belfast, Northern Ireland: DHSSPS.

Foley, G., & Gentile, J. 2010. Non-verbal communication in psychotherapy. *Psychiatry*, 7(6): 38–44.

Hogan, D.B., Bailey, P., Black, S., Carswell, A., Chertkow, H., & Clarke, B. 2008. Diagnosis and treatment of dementia: 5. Nonpharmacologic and pharmacologic therapy for mild to moderate dementia. *Canadian Medical Association Journal*, 179(10): 1019–1026.

Kitwood, T. 1997. *Dementia Reconsidered*. Maidenhead, UK: Open University Press.

Knott, D. 2012. From communication skills to psychological interventions. In *Psychological Interventions*, edited by Smith, G., 25–36. Maidenhead, UK: Open University Press.

Mast, B. 2014. Whole person assessment and care planning. In *Excellence in Dementia Care*, 2nd edition, edited by Downs, M., & Bowers, B., 290–302. Maidenhead, UK: Open University Press.

Moniz-Cook, E., & Manthorpe, J. (Editors). 2009. *Early Psychological Interventions in Dementia: Evidence-Based Practice*. London: Kingsley.

National Collaborating Centre for Mental Health. 2007—Updated 2011. *Dementia: A NICE-SCIE Guideline on Supporting People with Dementia and Their Carers in Health and Social Care*. National Clinical Practice Guideline Number 42. Leicester, UK: British Psychological Society and Gaskell.

Nursing and Midwifery Council. (2010) *Standards for Pre-registration Nursing Education*. London: Nursing and Midwifery Council.

O'Carroll, M., & Park, A. 2007. *Essential Mental Health Nursing Skills*. London: Mosby.

Orgeta, V., Qazi, A., Spector, A., & Orrell, M. 2014. Psychological treatments for depression and anxiety in dementia and mild cognitive impairment. *Cochrane Database of Systematic Reviews*, (1). doi:10.1002/14651858.CD009125.pub2.

Oyebode, J., & Clare, L. 2014. Supporting cognitive abilities. In *Excellence in Dementia Care*, 2nd edition, edited by Downs, M., & Bowers, B., 189–202. Maidenhead, UK: Open University Press.

Parker, D. 2012. Psychological interventions and working with the older adult. In *Psychological Interventions*, edited by Smith, G., 120–132. Maidenhead, UK: Open University Press.

Paukert, A.L., Calleo, J., Kraus-Schuman, C., Snow, L., Wilson, N., Petersen, N.J., Kunik, M.E., & Stanley, M.A. 2010. Peaceful Mind: An open trial of cognitive-behavioral therapy for anxiety in persons with dementia. *International Psychogeriatrics*, 22(6): 1012–1021.

Rigby, P., & Alexander, J. 2008. Building positive therapeutic relationships. In *Fundamental Aspects of Mental Health Nursing*, edited by Dooher, J., 103–116. London: Quay Books.

Scottish Government. 2013. *Scotland's National Dementia Strategy: 2013–2016*. Edinburgh: Scottish Government.

Smith, G. 2012. An introduction to psychological interventions. In *Psychological Interventions*, edited by Smith, G., 1–10. Maidenhead, UK: Open University Press.

Smith, G. 2014. *Mental Health Nursing at a Glance*. Chichester, UK: Wiley Blackwell.

Van Zadelhoff, E., Verbeek, H., Widdershoven, G., Van Rossum, E., & Abma, T. 2011. Good care in group home living for people with dementia. Experiences of residents, family and nursing staff. *Journal of Clinical Nursing*, 20: 2490–2500.

Welsh Assembly Government. 2011. *National Dementia Vision for Wales*. Cardiff, Wales: Welsh Assembly Government.

Woods, L. 2012. Psychological interventions in anxiety and depression. In *Psychological Interventions*, edited by Smith, G., 51–64. Maidenhead, UK: Open University Press.

World Health Organisation. 2012. *Dementia: A Public Health Priority*. Geneva, Switzerland: World Health Organisation.

Zarit, S.H., & Zarit, J.M. 2014. Supporting families coping with dementia: flexibility and change. In *Excellence in Dementia Care*, 2nd edition, edited by Downs, M., & Bowers, B., 176–188. Maidenhead, UK: Open University Press.

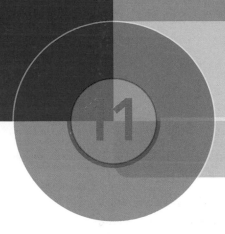

Technological approaches

11

GRAHAME SMITH AND DENISE PARKER

AIM

- To explore technological approaches used in dementia care

OBJECTIVES

- Critically reflect on the use of assistive technology as a way of supporting dementia care
- Recognise what is meant by the terms *telehealth* and *telecare*
- Appreciate how innovation can be framed as a user-led process
- Consider co-creation as a structured person-centred process

OVERVIEW

The United Kingdom is currently the leading European nation in the adoption of telecare, with 1.7 million current users, spending £106 million in 2010. United Kingdom spending on telecare in 2015 is projected to be £251 million. (Gibson et al., 2014: 2)

With the concern that there will be a potential increase in demand for dementia care services globally, there has been an increasing drive to develop innovative and cost-effective ways to deliver services now and in the future (Woods et al., 2013; World Health Organisation, 2012; Roe, 2007). At the forefront of this drive is the increasing use of technology. For this technology to be cost effective it has to improve the quality of care for people living with dementia and it has to meet their real needs (Department of Health, 2011). Crucial to this approach are ensuring that care underpinned by technology is person centred and that people with dementia are supported to function as independently as possible (Woods et al., 2013; Kitwood, 1997). This in itself is a challenge—even with a move towards personalised care, people living with dementia still report that their needs are not being fully met. The increasing use of technology may be one way of addressing this issue (Dröes et al., 2006; Nugent, 2007; Lauriks et al., 2007):

> Advances in computing technologies, telecommunications and the widespread prevalence and uptake of the Internet have offered a completely new paradigm to the way in which care can be provided. (Nugent, 2007: 473)

Generally the use of technology within the dementia care field is perceived as beneficial, especially where it compensates for cognitive impairment or maintains cognitive function (Lauriks et al., 2007; Nugent, 2007; Mate-Kole et al., 2007). Technology can be used to promote social interaction, help promote activities of daily living, and enable memory. The types of technology include email, online social networking, and portable information and communication technology (ICT) devices that prompt memory (Nugent, 2007; Lauriks et al., 2007; Oriani et al., 2004). Taking increased use of technology into consideration, this chapter looks at how technology is used within the care delivery process. It also considers how people living with dementia can co-create their own technological solutions (Woods et al., 2013). A scenario-based approach is used throughout to pragmatically explore the issues:

Clair has worked as a practitioner within the dementia care field for over 20 years. Recently Clair attended a conference where it was mentioned that 'apps' were being used as memory-enabling tools for people living with dementia. On further investigation Clair found that another National Health Services (NHS) Trust within the local area was using these apps as an integrated care package approach for people recently diagnosed with early-stage dementia. After spending time liaising with this service Clair was keen that her service consider using a similar approach.

ASSISTIVE TECHNOLOGY

As we know, assistive technologies are being increasingly used within the care delivered to people with dementia. As practitioners we are not always sure what is and is not an assistive technology, which can be defined as follows (Gibson et al., 2014):

> A catch-all term for 'any device or system that allows an individual to perform a task that they would otherwise be unable to do, or increases the ease and safety with which the task can be performed' (Royal Commission on Long Term Care, 1999). Does not only refer to electronic equipment; can refer to quite simple devices such as calendar clocks, products providing assistance with activities of daily living, devices which promote activity and enjoyment. (p. 2)

Generally practitioners view assistive technologies as either telehealth or telecare. We explore these technologies further in the next two sections (Gibson et al., 2014). This chapter takes a broad view of assistive technologies, and due to the ever-changing technological landscape there is no attempt to define what is and is not an assistive technology. Rather, this chapter explores how assistive technology in its broadest sense can enable living with dementia to have a good quality of life (Woods et al., 2013; Gibson et al., 2014). There are a number of challenges for practitioners using or wanting to use assistive technologies. One of these challenges is that carers generally perceive assistive technology as beneficial, but only if they are comfortable using technology in general and have had training in how to use assistive technology (Torp et al., 2008; Lauriks et al., 2007; Engstrom et al., 2006; Landau et al., 2009; Rialle et al., 2008). Another challenge is that assistive technologies are not routinely 'co-created' with people with dementia. This lack of real-life testing may mean that the assistive technology does not meet the real-life needs of the users. It also may mean that it stands apart from the other care the person with dementia is receiving (Woods et al., 2013; Lauriks et al., 2007; Topo, 2009; Carswell et al., 2009; Kolanowski & Whall, 2000; McCullagh et al., 2009; Prince et al., 2009).

The potential of assistive technology is that it could help to safely support a person with dementia to stay at home longer by delaying the move to residential care as long as risk dictates. This managed delay could also reduce the problems associated with this dramatic change (Woods et al., 2013; Manthorpe, 2009). Simple solutions, not always technological (e.g. improved lighting, bath aids, memory prompts, alarms, and improving the layout of the home environment) can also reduce risk and in turn increase the autonomy of people with dementia (Woods et al., 2013; Dementia Services Development Centre, 2007). Let us return to Clair:

Clair's line manager has agreed that the service could look at using a memory-enabling app. On this basis, Clair has been asked to write a proposal. To make sense of this confusing field Clair has started to think about the following (Gibson et al., 2014):

- Will the app be used by a person with dementia technology designed specifically for that person?
- Will the app be used by other people as well? Is it interactive?
- Will the app be solely designed for the carer to keep the person with dementia safe?

TELEHEALTH AND TELECARE

Telehealth can be defined as

> … a subtype of AT including technology-supported medical or nursing tasks undertaken in a person's home or other remote site, especially sending biometric data from the patient to the health care system and/or sending advice, instructions or reminders from the health care system to the patient. (Gibson et al., 2014)

and telecare as

> … a subtype of AT which usually involves the remote monitoring of people living in their own homes, communicating with them at a distance via telephony and the internet. Devices used to facilitate independence and enhance personal safety. Telecare includes community alarms, sensors and movement detectors, and the use of video conferencing to communicate with carers. (Gibson et al., 2014: 2)

Most health and social care practitioners working with people living with dementia will more likely use telecare rather than telehealth for keeping people safe and for remote monitoring of physical symptoms (Gibson et al., 2014; Woods et al., 2013). Telehealth will be more commonly used where comorbidity with a long-term physical condition, such as chronic obstructive pulmonary disease (COPD) exists (Woods et al., 2013). Telecare systems or devices work by using sensors to monitor for emergencies or daily life changes that are connected with risk such as leaving the gas cooker on or going for a walk in the middle of the night alone (Woods et al., 2013). The system is usually linked to a designated person or a call centre, and when a concern is raised the informal or formal caregiver is notified along with individuals at other services if required (Woods et al., 2013; Gibson et al., 2014). Alarms can be provided without them being linked to a telecare service, according to Gibson et al. (2014), within the UK,

> Almost all local authorities provided community alarms, with 196 of these also offering telecare, either integrated into community alarm services or provided through a separate local entity. A small minority of local authorities (48) provided community alarms but no telecare service, although many of these also indicated that they hoped to provide telecare in the near future. (Gibson et al., 2014: 11)

The focus of telecare is to keep people with dementia safe while enabling them to be independent within their own home or other community setting as long as possible (Gibson et al., 2014; Woods et al., 2013). A telecare service is a preventative measure, and it can also promote a sense of security. The use of telecare services is rapidly expanding. On this basis, there is a need for more research and evaluation in this area, especially related to its potential to promote and increase independent living (Gibson et al., 2014; Woods et al., 2013). A growth area is the integrated use of telecare and telehealth in a 'smart home'—a home that can seamlessly monitor a person's activities within the home and respond accordingly through such devices as alarms and reminders. The application of this type of approach is still in the early stages (Gibson et al., 2014; Woods et al., 2013; Martin et al., 2008; Bath Institute of Medical Engineering, 2009).

Smart home approaches help maintain existing levels of independence. They aid people with dementia to remain longer in their own homes and they can assist in the management of challenging behaviour within the home setting, such as night wandering (Woods et al., 2013; Martin et al., 2008; Evans et al., 2007). To receive telecare and telehealth, a person living with dementia will be assessed both financially and in terms of their day-to-day functioning levels (Gibson et al., 2014; Hagen et al., 2004). Considering the 'functioning' part of the assessment process, let us return to Clair:

Clair, working with the multidisciplinary team, has started to think about the factors that should be considered when determining the use of the memory-enabling app as an assistive technology. These will include the following (Hagen et al., 2004: 285–286):

1. The person with dementia:
   - Diagnosis
   - Severity, nature and duration of the condition
   - Other health-related conditions
   - Psychosocial functioning

2. The carer:
   - The nature of their caring role
   - Motivation and skills in the use of assistive technology
3. The environment:
   - Nature and extent of health and social care service provided
   - Description of the home environment
4. The app:
   - Design
   - Function
   - Reliability

INNOVATION

Before creating an app as an assistive technology the designer has to decide what the device would be used for. Gibson et al. (2014) categorise the use of assistive technology in the following ways:

1. Devices used 'by' people with dementia. These were devices that could be used independently by the person with dementia and were usually supportive and responsive products which helped people in completing their everyday activities in some way, by making activities easier (e.g. medication dispensers), by providing prompts (memory aids; simple signage) or by raising alerts (e.g. reminder alarms).
2. Devices used 'with' people with dementia. These were collaborative devices which fostered interaction between a person with dementia and other people or between the person and the technology. In most cases these devices encouraged, supported or enabled communication (e.g. reminiscence aids), or helped a person engage with others through interactive forms of 'play' (e.g. puzzles and games, sensory play).
3. Devices used 'on' people with dementia. These devices could intervene in some way in a person's life, but operated without the active or direct participation of the person with dementia. Such products could monitor people's movements or activities, alerting a carer or tele-operator in an emergency (e.g. telecare), could give quick access to a person (e.g. keysafes) or could lessen or prevent the risk of harm from individual (e.g. fall detectors), internal (e.g. gas or smoke alarms) or external sources (e.g. telephone blockers). Although not exclusively so, the majority of these products sought to manage, lessen or mitigate risks to the person with dementia receiving them. (Gibson et al., 2014: 6–7)

You would expect a memory-enabling app to be used by and with people with dementia. The aim would be to enhance a person's cognitive abilities in the hope that you enable the person to continue to function independently (Woods et al., 2013; Kerr, Cunningham, & Martin, 2010). The app would be a compensatory strategy, one of many within a person's integrated care package. It would be uploaded onto a mobile phone or a similar personal device (Woods et al., 2013; Kerr, Cunningham, & Martin, 2010). Developing an app to be used as a means of enabling memory that could potentially improve the quality of care outcomes for people living with dementia can be viewed as being innovative (Woods et al., 2013; Department of Health, 2011).

For this approach to work and to address real needs, it is vital people living with the everyday challenges of dementia are central to the innovation process (Woods et al., 2013; Richardson & Cotton, 2011; Weber, 2011). A person-centred approach to innovation is fundamental, especially where the intention is for the app to be part of the care delivery process (Kitwood, 1997; Richardson & Cotton, 2011; Department of Health, 2011). This way of working requires the practitioner to think about people with dementia in terms of their strengths rather than their deficits. On this basis, the app should be

> … designed based upon the strengths and desires of the person and not upon his/her deficits, in order to stimulate the user and promote autonomous activity. … The best long-term outcome might not be the one which provides the highest level of compensation but instead makes the most use of these preserved abilities. (Pino et al., 2013: 1251)

Designing for strengths rather than focusing on deficits should not be an unusual way of working for the practitioner, as a strengths-based approach to managing risk (positive risk management) is a common enough approach within dementia care settings (Smith, 2014; Rylance & Simpson, 2012). You can see the similarities in the following view:

> Positive risk management means engaging with the service user and others involved in their care at every stage, as well as recognizing and building on the resources the service user already has available to them, including their own strengths and coping strategies. It also needs to be acknowledged that people have the right to make choices and that sometimes those choices may involve a degree of risk. (Rylance & Simpson, 2012: 17)

Increasingly, people are using technology to enhance their lives. People with dementia should not be treated in a way that prevents them being afforded the opportunity to develop and use technology that has the potential to assist them in maintaining their independence (Woods et al., 2013; Kerr, Cunningham, & Martin, 2010; Ham, Dixon, & Brooke, 2012; Pino et al., 2013). Returning to Clair:

Before Clair presents her proposal she needs to define innovation within a health and social care context. On this basis Clair had initially decided to use the following definition:

> Innovation in healthcare is defined as those changes that help healthcare practitioners focus on the patient by helping healthcare professionals work smarter, faster, better and more cost effectively. (Thakur, Hsu, & Fontenot, 2012: 564)

However she felt it was not person centred so she decided to use the following:

> User-driven innovation is defined as 'the process of tapping users' knowledge in order to develop new products, services and concepts. A user-driven innovation process is based on an understanding of true user needs and a systematic involvement of users'. (Bjørkquist, Ramsdal, & Ramsdal, 2015: 4)

Adding to this definition Clair was keen that people living with dementia were involved in the implementation of the app at the level at which

… the recipient of services participates and significantly influences decisions either within a very wide framework of options or with no limitations—where the service provider does not make the decisions but only executes the consumer's decisions. (Bjørkquist, Ramsdal, & Ramsdal, 2015: 5)

CO-CREATION

Person-centred dementia care and user-driven innovation are processes that have similar aims. The user is the focal point of the process. These approaches are also highly compatible when innovating (Woods et al., 2013). The innovation process within health and social care needs to have structure. A starting place in the design of this structure is to identify key partners and then identify how the collaborative process will be managed to guarantee successful outcomes.

The triple-helix approach is a way of structuring collaborative innovation. Interested parties from academia, business, and the health and social care sector are brought together to innovate (Etzkowitz & Leydesdorff, 1997). One of the limitations of this approach is that it does not refer directly to the user—in this case people living with dementia. When users are directly involved, driving the innovation process by focusing on their real-life needs, the approach is called the quadruple helix approach (Woods et al., 2013; Dewsbury & Linskell, 2011). The triple or quadruple helix can be used to create an open innovation group in which all interested parties innovate by exploring the everyday challenges of living with dementia with a focus on co-creating sustainable solutions that fit with the real needs of people living with dementia (Woods et al., 2013; Etzkowitz & Leydesdorff, 1997).

People living with dementia being treated as equal partners and in a person-centred manner is fundamental to this way of working, especially where there is a focus on improving care outcomes (Woods et al., 2013; Richardson & Cotton, 2011; Department of Health, 2011). The success of this approach is dependent on all partners listening to and engaging fully with each other (Weber, 2011; Dewsbury & Linskell, 2011). A principle of good co-creation, whether it is a service change or the development of a technological innovation, is to value the skills, knowledge, time and expertise of people living with dementia, and viewing them as experts. This should result in positive change (The King's Fund, 2012; Ham, Dixon, & Brooke, 2012). Valuing and listening are important, especially in the case of assistive technologies being generally criticised for not meeting the real needs of people with dementia (Woods et al., 2013; Lauriks et al., 2007). The design of assistive technology can tend to focus on the carer's needs rather than the needs of the person with dementia:

Typically, it is the caregiver who is the source of information in the design process … and people with dementia are not engaged directly. … Consequently, commercially available assistive technologies for people with dementia generally have a safety focus. When people with dementia are empowered through being given a voice in design, this has given rise to designs that address social interaction with others …, facilitate reminiscing about their past or that help the person with dementia maintain their autonomy through support for activities of daily living. (Lindsay et al., 2012: 522)

Co-creation will place people living with dementia in the centre of the process but for it to be effective—meaning that a proposed solution is owned by people with dementia not just their carers—the process needs to work with a real-life understanding of what it is like to live with dementia (Ståhlbröst & Bergvall-Kåreborn, 2011). One method of generating this understanding is to support people living with dementia to talk about their everyday challenges and while actively listening identify common themes which can be used to codesign a specific solution (Estey-Burtt & Baldwin, 2014; Bergvall-Kåreborn & Ståhlbröst, 2010).

Chapter 14 provides an example of how co-creation as a collaborative process underpinned by the quadruple helix can be further structured through the living lab approach. This approach is similar to action research; it is pragmatic, collaborative, and user centric (Bergvall-Kåreborn, Holst, & Ståhlbröst, 2009):

> Action research ... is a well suited methodology for the Living Lab, since both approaches emphasise interaction between theory and practice, involve many different stakeholders with distinct roles relevant in the situation, and highlight the importance of constant reflection in order to follow wherever the situation leads. (p. 4)

Using a structured approach to co-creation assists the practitioner in capturing the voice of people living with dementia. The next stage is cross-checking that the practitioner's understanding of the common themes is the same as all the partners, including people with dementia (Smith, 2012). By cross-checking, all voices are valued irrespective of whether the person is diagnosed with dementia. The practitioner in effect is being person centred (Parker, 2012). The practitioner also has to take into consideration that assistive technology is an intervention, and that it needs to be evidence based. On this basis, the practitioner will need to give equal weight to the evidence base and to the voice of people living with dementia (Smith, 2012; Estey-Burtt & Baldwin, 2014). A way of doing this is to adopt a multiple-meaning approach by which the practitioner works with both forms of evidence (Smith, 2012; Estey-Burtt & Baldwin, 2014; Johnson et al., 2007). Once the checking process is complete the practitioner can then work with all partners to start to consider potential solutions. The success of this phase is again dependent on all partners having an equal input (Weber, 2011). The value of people living with dementia being an equal partner in this phase is that the eventual solution is more likely to fit their real needs (Woods et al., 2013; Bergvall-Kåreborn & Ståhlbröst, 2010).

Overall the value of the co-creation process is that championing the real needs of people living with dementia increases the chances of developing sustainable solutions to these individuals' everyday challenges (Woods et al., 2013; Bergvall-Kåreborn, Holst, & Ståhlbröst, 2009; Estey-Burtt & Baldwin, 2014). This process also has a social value, according to Pallot and Pawar (2012): 'Co-creation is fuelled by aspirations for longer term, humanistic, and more sustainable ways of living' (p. 7). This is especially important in the dementia field, in which there is currently a societal drive to improve the quality of life of people living with dementia (Woods et al., 2013; Department of Health, 2009). Let us return to Clair:

Clair, influenced by the literature on living labs and co-creation, has decided in her proposal to recommend the following process (Bergvall-Kåreborn, Holst, & Ståhlbröst, 2009):

- Plan the project and build the project team, including people living with dementia
- Identify needs and prioritise through agreement on common themes
- Identify potential solutions and then test and evaluate, including memory-enabling technology already being used

---

CHAPTER SUMMARY

Globally the increasing use of assistive technology is being driven by the concern that there will be a potential increase in demand for dementia care services. A widely held view is that the use of these technologies will help in the development of more cost-effective ways to deliver services now and in the future.

Practitioners are not always sure what is and is not an assistive technology, especially as it is used as a 'catchall' term. There are a number of challenges for practitioners using assistive technologies; people living with dementia need to be given training in how to use these technologies, and it is important to recognise assistive technologies that are 'off the shelf' and not co-created may not meet the real-life needs of people living with dementia.

Assistive technologies must be 'strengths based' with a focus on enabling people living with dementia to live well. Also, to meet real needs, the innovation process should be user driven. In addition, an emphasis should be placed on understanding the 'true needs' of people living with dementia.

Co-creation is a structured process that systematically places people living with dementia in the centre of the design process. It should work actively with a true understanding of what it is like to live with dementia. This understanding is generated through supporting people living with dementia to talk about their everyday challenges with a focus on the practitioner actively listening and then facilitating the journey towards discovering potential solutions.

REFLECTION ON LEARNING

1. What must assistive technology improve?
2. Define assistive technologies.
3. What is the difference between a telehealth device and a telecare device?
4. What must the practitioner consider during the assistive technology assessment process?
5. Describe the three uses of assistive technology.
6. Describe user-driven innovation.
7. What is the triple-helix process?
8. Why is the term *quadruple helix* preferable in the dementia field?
9. What is a living lab? (see Chapter 14)
10. What else in addition to evidence based does assistive technology need to be?

REFERENCES

Bath Institute of Medical Engineering. 2009. Smart Way of Living for People with Dementia. http://www.bath.ac.uk/ news/2007/1/24/smarthouse.html.

Bergvall-Kåreborn, B., Holst, M., & Ståhlbröst. 2009. Concept Design with a Living Lab Approach. Paper presented at the 42nd International Conference on System Sciences, Hawaii, May.

Bjørkquist, C., Ramsdal, H., & Ramsdal, K. 2015. User participation and stakeholder involvement in health care innovation—Does it matter? *European Journal of Innovation Management*, 18(1): 2–18.

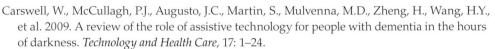

Carswell, W., McCullagh, P.J., Augusto, J.C., Martin, S., Mulvenna, M.D., Zheng, H., Wang, H.Y., et al. 2009. A review of the role of assistive technology for people with dementia in the hours of darkness. *Technology and Health Care*, 17: 1–24.

Dementia Services Development Centre. 2007. *Best Practice in Design for People with Dementia*. Stirling, UK: Dementia Services Development Centre.

Department of Health. 2009. *Living Well with Dementia: A National Dementia Strategy*. London: Department of Health.

Department of Health. 2011. *NHS Operating Framework 2012–13*. London: Department of Health.

Dewsbury, G., & Linskell, J. 2011. Smart home technology for safety and functional independence: The UK experience. *NeuroRehabilitation*, 28(3): 249–260.

Dröes, R.-M., Boelens-Van Der Knoop, E.C.C., Bos, J., Teake, L.M., Ettema, P., Gerritsen, D.L., Hoogeveen, F., De Lange, J., & SchöLzel-Dorenbos, C.J.M. 2006. Quality of life in dementia in perspective: An explorative study of variations in opinions among people with dementia and their professional caregivers, and in literature. *Dementia*, 5(4): 533–558.

Engstrom, M., Lindqvist, R., Ljunggren, B., & Carlsson, M. 2006. Relatives' opinions of IT support, perceptions of irritations and life satisfaction in dementia care. *Journal of Telemedicine and Telecare*, 12(5): 246–250.

Estey-Burtt, B., & Baldwin, C. 2014. Ethics in dementia care: storied lives, storied ethics. In *Excellence in Dementia Care*, 2nd edition, edited by Downs, M., & Bowers, B., 53–65. Maidenhead, UK: Open University Press.

Etzkowitz, H., & Leydesdorff, L. (Editors). 1997. *Universities in the Global Knowledge Economy: A Triple Helix of University-Industry-Government Relations*. London: Cassell.

Evans, N., Orpwood, R., Adlam, T., & Chad, J. 2007. Evaluation of an enabling smart flat for people with dementia. *Journal of Dementia Care*, 15: 33–37.

Gibson, G., Newton, L., Pritchard, G., Finch, T., Brittain, K., & Robinson, L. 2014. The provision of assistive technology products and services for people with dementia in the United Kingdom. *Dementia*, 0(0): 1–21. doi:10.1177/1471301214532643.

Hagen, I., Holthe, T., Gilliard, J., Topo, P., Cahill, S., Begley, E., Jones, K., et al. 2004. Development of a protocol for the assessment of assistive aids for people with dementia. *Dementia*, 3(3): 281–296.

Ham, C., Dixon, A., & Brooke, B. 2012. *Transforming the Delivery of Health and Social Care*. London: Kings Fund.

Kerr, D., Cunningham, C., & Martin, S. 2010. *Telecare and Dementia: Using Telecare Effectively in the Support of People with Dementia*. Stirling, UK: University of Stirling, Dementia Services Development Centre.

The King's Fund. 2012. Experience-Based Co-Design Toolkit: Working with Patients to Improve Health Care. The King's Fund website. http://www.kingsfund.org.uk/projects/ebcd.

Kitwood, T. 1997. *Dementia Reconsidered*. London: Open University Press.

Kolanowski, A.M., & Whall, A.L. 2000. Toward holistic theory-based intervention for dementia behaviour. *Holistic Nursing Practice*, 14(2): 67–76.

Landau, R., Werner, S., Auslander, G.K., Shoval, N., & Heinik, J. 2009. Attitudes of family and professional care-givers towards the use of GPS for tracking patients with dementia: An exploratory study. *British Journal of Social Work*, 39(4): 670–692.

Lauriks, S., Reinersmann, A., Van der Roest, H.G., Meiland, F.J., Davies, R.J., Moelaert, F., Mulvenna, M.D., Nugent, C.D., & Droes, R.M. 2007. Review of ICT-based services for identified unmet needs in people with dementia. *Ageing Research Reviews*, 6(3): 223–246.

Lindsay, S., Brittain, K., Jackson, D., Ladha, C., Ladha, K., & Olivier, P. 2012. Empathy, participatory design and people with dementia. In *Proceedings of the SIGCHI Conference on Human Factors in Computing Systems*, 521–530, general chair Konstan, J.A. New York: ACM.

Manthorpe, J. 2009. Decisions, decisions … linking personalization to person-centred care. In *Decision-Making, Personhood and Dementia: Exploring the Interface*, edited by O'Connor, D., & Purves, B., 91–105. London: Kingsley.

Martin, S., Kelly, G., Kernohan, W.G., Mcleight, B., & Nugent, C. 2008. Smart home technologies for health and social care. *Cochrane Database of Systematic Reviews*, 4. doi:10.1002/14651858.CD006412.pub2.

Mate-Kole, C.C., Fellows, R.P., Said, P.C., McDougal, J., Catayong, K., & Dang, V. 2007. Use of computer assisted and interactive cognitive training programs with moderate to severely demented individuals: A preliminary study. *Ageing & Mental Health*, 11(5): 483–493.

McCullagh, P.J., Carswell, W., Augusto, J.C., Martin, S., Mulvenna, M.D., Zheng, H., Wang, H.Y., et al. 2009. State of the Art on Night-Time Care of People with Dementia. Paper presented at the IET Assisted Living Conference, London, March.

Nugent, C.D. 2007. Editorial: ICT in the elderly and dementia. *Aging & Mental Health*, 11(5): 473–476.

Oriani, M., Moniz-Cook, E., Binetti, G., Zanieri, G., Frisoni, G.B., Geroldi, C., De Vreese, L.P., & Zanetti, O. 2004. An electronic memory aid to support prospective memory in patients in the early stages of Alzheimer's disease: A pilot study. *Aging & Mental Health*, 7: 22–27.

Pallot, M., & Pawar, K. 2012. A Holistic Model of User Experience for Living Lab Experiential Design. Paper presented at the Engineering, Technology and Innovation 18th International ICE Conference, Munich, June.

Parker, D. 2012. Psychological interventions and working with the older adult. In *Psychological Interventions*, edited by Smith, G., 120–131. Maidenhead, UK: Open University Press.

Pino, M., Benveniste, S., Rigaud, A., & Jouen, F. 2013. Key factors for a framework supporting the design, provision, and assessment of assistive technology for dementia care. *Assistive Technology Research Series*, 33: 1247–1252.

Prince, M.J., Acosta, D., Castro-Costa, E., Jackson, J., & Shaji, K.S. 2009. Packages of care for dementia in low- and middle-income countries. *PLoS Med*, 6(11): e1000176. doi:10.1371/journal.pmed.1000176.

Rialle, V., Ollivet, C., Guigui, C., & Herve, C. 2008. What do family caregivers of Alzheimer's disease patients desire in smart home technologies? Contrasted results of a wide survey. *Methods of Information in Medicine*, 47(1): 63–69.

Richardson, A., & Cotton, R. 2011. *No Health without Mental Health: Developing an Outcomes Based Approach*. London: NHS Confederation.

Roe, P.R.W. (Editor). 2007. *Towards an Inclusive Future: Impact and Wider Potential of Information and Communication Technologies*. Brussels, Belgium: COST.

Royal Commission on Long Term Care. 1999. *With Respect to Old Age: Long Term Care—Rights and Responsibilities*. London: Department of Health.

Rylance, R., & Simpson, P. 2012. Psychological interventions and managing risk. In *Psychological Interventions in Mental Health Nursing*, edited by Smith, G., 11–23. Maidenhead, UK: Open University Press.

Smith, G. 2012. An introduction to psychological interventions. In *Psychological Interventions*, edited by Smith, G., 1–10. Maidenhead, UK: Open University Press.

Smith, G. 2014. *Mental Health Nursing at a Glance*. Chichester, UK: Wiley Blackwell.

Thakur, R., Hsu, S.H.Y., & Fontenot, G. 2012. Innovation in healthcare: Issues and future trends. *Journal of Business Research*, 65: 562–569.

Topo, P. 2009. Technology studies to meet the needs of people with dementia and their caregivers: A literature review. *Journal of Applied Gerontology*, 28(1): 5–37.

Torp, S., Hanson, E., Hauge, S., Ulstein, I., & Magnusson, L. 2008. A pilot study of how information and communication technology may contribute to health promotion among elderly spousal carers in Norway. *Health and Social Care in the Community*, 16(1): 75–85.

Weber, M.E.A. 2011. *Customer Co-Creation in Innovations: A Protocol for Innovating with End Users*. Eindhoven, the Netherlands: Eindhoven University of Technology.

Woods, L., Smith, G., Pendleton, J., & Parker, D. 2013. *Innovate Dementia Baseline Report: Shaping the Future for People Living with Dementia*. Liverpool, UK: Liverpool John Moores University.

World Health Organisation. 2012. *Dementia: A Public Health Priority*. Geneva, Switzerland: World Health Organisation.

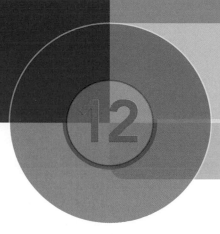

The environment

DENISE PARKER AND ROBERT G. MACDONALD

AIM

- To consider the environment as a key mediating factor in supporting people to live well with dementia

OBJECTIVES

- To recognise that people with dementia have a right to age in place in a safe and secure environment
- To reflect on the role of supported housing
- To appreciate that an environment can be dementia friendly
- To identify the key principles of a good care environment

OVERVIEW

To design dementia-friendly dwellings and environments of the future, at different stages of dementia we need to work in collaboration with many people. We need professional teams of architects, landscape designers, technologists, museum and galleries workers, interior designers, product manufacturers, clinical nursing and medical psychological staff—in fact, we need a "living lab" and a whole range and cross section of skills. This inclusive design process should set out to enable the voices of people living with dementia to speak about their environment in design terms (Woods et al., 2013).

The care of people living with dementia has traditionally been firmly grounded in the medical model. This included 'warehousing' of people living with dementia (society still colludes in warehousing on an industrial scale). This involves needs of the person living with dementia being met, as regards our traditional notion of the needs of people living with dementia, namely physical needs, particularly when dementia is advanced, and progressing to 'total nursing care'. The focus here is on what we do 'to' people with dementia. The interventions that we use have traditionally focused on basic physiological needs, rather than psychological needs. We have been realising that the best people to inform services, governments and businesses about the needs of people with dementia are the 'experts by experience', namely the people living with dementia and their caregivers (Woods et al., 2013). We still have a long way to go. By considering the environment in the mix of unmet needs, the net is widening to involve the community in helping to meet those needs in part. In 2002, a groundbreaking document, *Forget Me Not*, published by the Audit Commission (2002), highlighted the lack of awareness about dementia among general practitioners. It has taken a national dementia strategy (Department of Health [DH], 2009) and dementia being made a Commissioning for Quality and Innovation (CQUIN) target (NHS [National Health Service] England, 2014)—a target whereby a standard needs to be met and only then is payment given—for us to be compelled as a society to see dementia as 'everybody's business'. In addition there has been a rallying call by Prime Minister David Cameron (DH, 2012) which states the need for dementia-friendly communities. This was built upon in the *Prime Minister's Challenge on Dementia 2020* (DH, 2015b). Davis et al. (2009) argue that we should reframe dementia as experience rather than a condition. This helps us to understand the person in the context of the residential environment.

In the 1980s and 1990s, there was a quiet revolution, led by Tom Kitwood, promoting the concept of 'personhood' as regards people living with dementia (Kitwood, 1997). In 1998, Loveday, Kitwood, and Bowe (1998) set out the basic rights of people with dementia receiving care. The Mental Capacity Act (2005) mentioned some of the ideas that are now familiar to us—notably the suggestion of people with dementia having the same rights as their fellow citizens. Kitwood's (1997) commentary on 'Malignant Social Psychology' indicates how it is that people caring for people living with dementia and society, rather than improving the situation and promoting independence, actually stifle growth and shatter self-esteem. The environment could be recognised as a contributing factor to malignant social psychology. If we agree that people living with dementia have the same rights as other citizens, then it follows that they also have the right to be a part of the community, and as much as possible, contribute to it regardless of whether they dwell in their own home or in a group setting. As human beings, our functioning can be seen as being due to our biological, physical and social resources and environmental characteristics.

Zeisel et al. (2003) indicated the link between behaviour and specific design features. They stated the potential role that the environment has to contribute to improvements in Alzheimer's symptoms, helping the person to understand, feel safe and be comforted by the environment. Person-centred care is integral to good dementia care (National Institute for Health and Clinical Excellence/Social Care Institute for Excellence Guidance [NICE/SCIE], 2006; DH, 2009).

> Sheltered accommodation is just that. Living in a project is sheltered from the big bad world and it provides a 24/7 environment within which safety needs and emotional support can be given to help self-growth of people with a mental illness. (Ellerby, 2013: 2)

Ellerby wrote from firsthand experience of psychosis. He eloquently stated what it is like for someone with a mental health condition to live in sheltered accommodation and the strengths of this. It is not unrealistic to link this to the case of people living with dementia.

Several aspects pertaining to dementia care and the environment have emerged as crucial to 'living well' with dementia rather than 'suffering from' dementia. These concepts relate to contemporary ethical care of people living with , and potentially developing, dementia. These concepts include 'dementia-friendly communities', 'aging in place', and dementia-friendly hospitals and residential and nursing homes. Collectively, these are known as 'dementia-friendly environments'. The use of personhood as a basis for good dementia care is recognised globally (Brooker, 2015). Brooker also stated that maintaining personhood in people with dementia is a global challenge (therefore for the global community).

To explore the issues that are raised at a more practical level, this chapter develops and explores the following scenario:

Marjorie and Alex are a couple in their mid 60s. They have brought up their three children, two girls and a boy, in their suburban semi-detached house in a suburb of a northern city in the UK. Most of their friends, close family and activities are in the community. They are active in the local church and community centre. Marjorie had a 'mini-stroke' last year, and Alex's arthritis has worsened. Marjorie has just been diagnosed with vascular dementia (World Health Organisation, 2007). The couple are beginning to consider their future, and one thing is clear: They want to stay in their house. However, they are concerned that it is not suitable as it is for the future.

In addition, co-author Rob Macdonald provides a commentary from an architect's perspective.

AGING IN PLACE

It is recognized that staying in a familiar home environment in old age can mitigate the effects of aging and dementia, thereby contributing to 'aging well'. Wahl, Iwarsson, and Oswald (2012) describe a 'strong desire of old and very old people to 'age in place', remaining in their familiar home environment or an environment of their choice for as long as possible' (p. 2). Since the early twenty-first century, the focus has been on providing options for housing for older people in keeping with their right to age in place (Evans, Vallelly, & Croucher, 2014: 338). It is over 40 years since Lawton and Nahemow (1973) theorised that healthy aging involved the phenomenon of a person–environment (P–E) interaction. They linked this to ecology. They stress that it is in later life that people are more prone to be sensitive to the P–E dynamic. Their competence environment press model indicates the link between physical environment and disability and environmental press. The model cites the demand that the environment makes on the person, and competence refers to the person's ability to respond to these demands adaptively. Making adaptations and simplifying a person's environment in a systematic manner can be essential for enabling independence and coping in one's own home (Woods et al., 2013). Functional performance is due to the interactions between competence and environmental demand (Chappel & Cooke, 2012). Lawton was one of the first authors to acknowledge the role of the environment in caregiving situations. He stressed the importance of issues such as the environment outside of the home, in the neighbourhood, transport and the wider community (Lawton, 1977). Lawton's ecological model (1990) sees aging in place as a P–E phenomenon. Wahl, Iwarsson, and Oswald (2012) state that consensus exists in gerontological literature that aging well requires both personal and environmental resources. They argue that hitherto, the role of the immediate physical environment has been somewhat neglected.

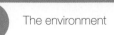

Returning to the chapter scenario:

Alex became increasingly worried about Marjorie's memory problems. Following her dementia diagnosis, they were given the chance to attend a 'postdiagnostic group' (DH, 2009) at the NHS Mental Health Trust hospital. They heard about advice for people living with dementia and their caregivers. They were asked to take part in a co-creation project to develop an app to help support people living with dementia to get through their day. As they already used a tablet computer, they agreed to take part in a European project called Innovate Dementia. They can see the benefit of such an app to help to maintain them in their present home environment. They were able to set alerts and messages for Marjorie to use when she was in the house alone. This looked helpful, as she was having difficulty sequencing when cooking and using instructions for the washing machine. She was able to read her own recipes, with photo instructions, and also do the same with her own appliances.

Technological solutions play a role in dementia care and in aging in place. In the chapter scenario, Alex and Marjorie are seeing the value of technology. Later, to maintain independence, they will have telecare and telehealth technology, such as 'Lifeline' sensors and alerts, and fall monitors. The use of assistive technology for people living with dementia is recognised and recommended as a part of care (NHS England, 2014).

Unfortunately, this would not be in their family home, as it proved not to be the most 'fit-for-purpose' environment. It would have been helpful had their house been built with the future in mind. In the 1940s, when their house was built, such issues were not in vogue. Life expectancy was not as high as later in the century. The main causes of death were infectious diseases, which often took people before very old age. Let us return to the scenario:

Marjorie and Alex spent a couple more years in their family home. However, without extensive adaptations, such as a downstairs toilet, a wet room, and access to the garden, the home is unsuitable. Fewer steps up to the front door would make a big difference also. Despite handrails, the risk of falling is a concern. Alex's arthritis is getting worse, and Marjorie has become more dependent on him. He worries in case she goes out and he cannot keep up with her, and she gets lost. This is distressing for both of them. Alex himself has not had a bath for 6 months as he cannot get in the tub. He has been showering at his son's house once a week. His own shower is over the bathtub. He worries about Marjorie becoming stuck in the bathtub, unable to get out safely. He believes that if they get rid of the bathtub in favour of a shower cubicle that this may have an impact on the value of the house. Besides, they cannot afford it.

The following is an in vivo example of a cooperative model of environmental intervention in Liverpool related by co-author Robert MacDonald from his personal experience as an architect working on these projects in Liverpool.

The collaborative design model is based on The Fieldway Elderly Persons Housing Cooperative at Huyton. Here, 32 elderly people worked with Bill Halsall and Robert MacDonald in designing their own dwellings from overall layout to bathrooms and kitchens.

Fieldway and many Housing Cooperatives in Merseyside were created in 'reaco-design' workshops that enabled small groups of people to come up with ideas for dwellings, gardens, streets and environments. There is a very significant archive and record of this unique Liverpool approach to 'co-design' including actual built projects, including The Eldonian Village. (The Eldonian Village was a co-creation project whereby residents helped to design their own dwellings. It is seen as an example of good practice and inclusiveness.)

From an architect's perspective, Rob MacDonald makes the following points:

In a dementia-friendly dwelling, if possible, all ground floor thresholds need to be level. Front and back gardens should be accessible to garden sheds and small green houses. Enjoyable, legible green spaces. Gardens should be planted with small trees and shrubs that attract wild life. Spaces for small pets, such as dogs. There should be outdoor sitting spaces with individually designed seating. Sheltered conservatories and greenhouses should be orientated to sunlight allowing access for Vitamin D. Are bungalows best and if not possible, how should we adapt existing houses? Downstairs toilet, bath, shower as additional extension?

Bay windows and porches, views to street activities and gardens. Eating space related to garden. Safe/secure staircase with additional handrails. Improved lighting throughout. Floor wall finishes colour and texture. Workrooms, hobby space for therapeutic activities of craft and making. Stimulating music, a Snoozelon space.

Technology in the home should be provided. In The Smart House (MI Liverpool, 2013) based at Liverpool Museum, there are examples of technology, such as Supra Keysafe, fingerprint lock, video entry system with handset, bogus caller panic button, voice prompt with door contacts. Cook easy kitchen appliances that keep you safe, one cup kettle, induction hob, talking microwave, wireless smoke detector.

There are rest easy products to help you relax at home, a big switch and remote socket, easy to use mobile phone, talking album, video entry system with handset, carbon monoxide detector, touch screen control unit, Amie personal trigger, lifeline Vi home unit, big picture phone, big jack controller, easy to see universal remote control, voice recorder, passive infra-red detector, sleep easy fall detector, talking watch, epilepsy sensor, enuresis sensor kit, bed occupancy sensor, wash easy (see www.moreindependent.co.uk).

SUPPORTED HOUSING

'Access to supported housing that is inclusive of people with dementia' (DH, 2009: 48) is recommended by England's national dementia strategy. It is no surprise that the place where most of us would want to live is our own home, the place where we feel safe, secure and comfortable and that is familiar to us. In the future, thanks to concepts such as aging in place, dementia-friendly communities and more hospital at home and intermediate care will be more dementia-friendly. However, there is still a considerable way to go (Alzheimer's Society, 2015).

Returning to the scenario:

Alex and Marjorie have heard of a new sheltered housing scheme being built in the city, just outside the centre. It is an 'extra care housing' (ECH) scheme (Petch, 2014). Some of their friends are talking about it. It is a complex of 50 apartments being built and managed by the local housing trust. The scheme takes people from the age of 55 onwards. There are several options by which potential residents can access these apartments, which include either exchanging existing social housing to rent an apartment, part ownership, or purchasing an apartment. At this stage of their lives, taking into consideration the health challenges that they have, Alex and Marjorie decide to sell their house and buy an apartment in 'Cedar Fields'.

In 2009, Dutton reviewed the literature from 1998 to 2008 of ECH and people with dementia. She found that there was not a strong evidence base and there was a lack of rigour in the research, with few studies focussing on the characteristics, experiences and outcomes of residents with dementia. She went on to identify important outcomes for people with dementia in ECH (Dutton, 2009: pp. 101–102):

- Maximisation of dignity and independence
- Individualised activities and experiences that bring pleasure and a sense of accomplishment
- Effective communication
- Meaningful social interactions
- Ability to maintain meaningful relationships
- Person-centred care
- Freedom from pain and discomfort
- The ability to age in place
- The appropriateness, layout and appearance of the physical environment
- Access to health care and palliative care when needed.

DEMENTIA-FRIENDLY ENVIRONMENTS

The Dementia Action Alliance (DAA) developed a declaration (www.dementiaaction.org.uk) to ensure that public and political commitment to improving dementia care in England is translated into action. It acknowledges that public awareness of dementia is high but that there is a lack of understanding of the condition and how it affects people. The alliance consists of organisations such as NHS Trusts, local authorities, and charities which have undertaken to work together to improve the everyday lives of people living with dementia. 'The organisations signed up to this declaration call upon all families, communities and organisations to work with us to transform quality of life for the millions of people affected by dementia' (DAA, 2015: 2). People living with dementia are some of the most stigmatised and socially excluded members of the community (Alzheimer's Disease International, 2012). In fact, Objective vi of the DH (2011) *No Health without Mental Health* policy (which covers all ages) is that public attitudes toward mental illness will improve and that stigma will be reduced. Initiatives such as the Alzheimer's Society and Public Health England's 'Dementia Friends' aim to reduce stigma. This is a national programme aimed at changing the public's perception of dementia by raising awareness of what it is like to live with dementia and turning that knowledge into action. An example of this is via a television advertisement at peak time and training the public to become Dementia friends trained by 'Dementia Champions' (https://www.dementiafriends.org.uk/), the aim being to make 4 million Dementia Friends in businesses and communities by 2020. 'By developing Dementia Friendly Communities (backed up by information and communication technology [ICT]) and reduce stigma, we can help people remain part of their communities' (Brooker, 2015: 5). Let us return to the scenario:

Alex and Marjorie went on a shopping trip to the city centre. Marjorie had lost weight recently, and all of her trousers were ill fitting. They went into a major department store. Marjory went to the changing room to try trousers on, with support from Alex. The assistant told them that men could not go into the changing room. The solution was to take them home and return them if they were not suitable. They needed returning. Marjorie tried to return them while Alex was having a comfort break. There was a queue at the checkout. Marjorie was trying to explain to the checkout operator that she was trying to return the trousers. The assistant curtly told her that she needed to go to the customer services counter. The woman behind her in the queue was huffing loudly. Marjorie was confused and upset in the middle of the aisle when Alex found her. She was lost and could not make sense of the layout of the store. The signage was confusing to her. To make matters worse, she wanted to use the women's lavatory also and could not find it. She was distressed. She caught sight of people watching her. Nobody offered to help.

Despite the recognition that such artefacts as the neighbourhood, transport and the wider community (Lawton, 1977) play a role in healthy aging, the extolling of dementia-friendly communities is not a recent phenomenon (Joseph Rowntree Foundation, 2014). The embracing and assimilation of people with mental health problems has been evident in Geel in Belgium for over 700 years, in the form of community-integrated care (since the thirteenth century and continues to be so today) (Goldstein & Godemont, 2003). 'Throughout history, cities have always been sites of experiments in urban living' (MacDonald, 2014, p. 2).

Again from an architect's perspective, Rob MacDonald makes the following points about a dementia-friendly neighbourhood (this is in line with 'connectivity' in dementia care):

The neighbourhood might be based on a 'Garden Suburb' model. Cities need to be age friendly. Friendly streets are essential with clearly demarked pavements. On-street car parking should not be intrusive. Level surfaces with limited trips and lamp posts and good street lighting should be provided. Clear pavements of bin storage and recycling bin shelters and storage shelters for mobility vehicles are required. Nearby public green spaces with trees (trees in public and private spaces), a green environment and dog walking space should be available. Changing seasonal landscapes can be used as natural stimulation. Opportunities for safe water features in public spaces should be considered. Good access to public transport (buses and trains is needed, as are a nearby local medical facility and holistic health centre. Integrated library and reading clubs and access to places that give spiritual support are essential, as well as local shopping within a walkable distance, with a variety of shops.

THE CARE ENVIRONMENT

Around a third of people with dementia live in residential care. This group of people is more likely to have a hospital admission due to such conditions as urinary infections, pressure sores, and dehydration than their peers without dementia. A further two-thirds of people with dementia live at home (DH, 2015b). Many people living with dementia at some point reside in residential care, whether a residential facility or a nursing home, due to the progressive nature of the disease (Alzheimer's Australia, 2004). In fact, 'the design of facilities can play an important role in ensuring that quality of life of people with dementia living in residential facilities is maximised' (Alzheimer's Australia, 2004: 2). In turn, according to Robert Yeoh, president of Alzheimer's Australia: 'This will reduce the stress and anxiety felt by families and carers when facing the often difficult decisions around residential placement and will encourage carers to take up residential opportunities' (Alzheimer's Australia, 2004: 2).

When purchasing and organising accommodation for care of people with dementia, health and social care managers need to ensure the needs of residents (NICE/SCIE, 2006). In fact, legislation—the Equality Act (2010)—compels this. In addition, Davis, Byers, and Nay (2009) challenged us to see dementia in terms of experience rather than merely as a condition. There is general consensus about good design in dementia care (Alzheimer's Australia, 2004). Marshall (2001) undertook a literature review of good design principles, recommending that accommodation for care of older adults should have such attributes as maximising independence, compensating for disability, control and balance stimuli, helping with orientation and understanding, and improving self-esteem.

Early studies concentrated on single aspects of design in response to dealing with particular problems (Woods et al., 2013). Design principles for designing environments for people with dementia have been refined over time. There are now tools to evaluate the impact of the built environment on people with dementia, such as the Design for Dementia Audit Tool from the University of Stirling (Cunningham, Marshall, & McManus, 2008). A literature review by the DH (2015a: 23–36), cited 12 design principles. Factors such as cognitive, sensory and physical impairments of people with dementia have to be considered, including the following:

- Provide a safe environment (considered an overarching principle)
- Provide optimum levels of stimulation
- Provide optimum lighting and contrast
- Provide a non–institutional-scale environment
- Support orientation
- Support way-finding and navigation
- Provide access to nature and the outdoors
- Promote engagement with friends, relatives, and staff
- Provide good visibility and visual access
- Promote privacy, dignity and independence
- Provide physical and meaningful activities
- Support diet, nutrition and hydration

CHAPTER SUMMARY

Designing dementia-friendly environments of the future is a collaborative venture, driven by people living with dementia, supported by professional teams of architects, landscape designers, technologists, museums, galleries, interior designers, product manufacturers, clinical nursing and medical psychological staff.

Aging in place and staying in a familiar home environment can contribute to aging well with dementia. People with dementia want to remain in their home environment for as long as possible. If this is not possible, they should be provided with housing and living options that support them to live well with dementia. Housing such as ECH for people with dementia should maximise independence and enable effective communication.

There is a strong societal commitment to improve dementia care throughout society, including increasing the public's awareness about dementia. This commitment is driven by the concern that people living with dementia are some of the most stigmatised and socially excluded members of society.

If individuals with dementia live in residential care they are more likely to have a hospital admission, due to such conditions as urinary infections, pressure sores, and dehydration, than their peers without dementia. Care improvements need to be realised, including ensuring residential facilities are designed in way that they are fit for purpose and that they are safe.

REFLECTION ON LEARNING

1. Name the groundbreaking document published by the Audit Commission in 2002.
2. Who led the quiet revolution in the 1980s to 1990s?
3. What can a familiar home environment in old age mitigate against?
4. Who was one of the first authors to recognise the role of the environment in caregiving situations?
5. Describe three examples of technology used within a smart home.
6. Identify four important outcomes for people with dementia in ECH.
7. Which organisation developed and published a declaration for dementia?
8. What should on-street car parking not be?
9. How many people with dementia live in residential care?
10. Describe 8 of the 12 design principles.

REFERENCES

Alzheimer's Australia. 2004. *Dementia and the Built Environment: Position Paper 3*. NSW Australia: Alzheimer's Australia.

Alzheimer's Disease International. 2012. *Overcoming the Stigma of Dementia*. London: Alzheimer's Disease International.

Alzheimer's Society. 2009. *Counting the Cost. Caring for People with Dementia on Hospital Wards*. London: Alzheimer's Society.

Alzheimer's Society. 2014. *Dementia 2014: Opportunity for Change*. London: Alzheimer's Society.

Alzheimer's Society. 2015. Dementia Friends. https://www.dementiafriends.org.uk/.

Audit Commission. 2002. *Forget Me Not 2002: Developing Mental Health Services for Older People*. London: Audit Commission.

Brooker, D. 2015. *Global Action in Personhood in Dementia*. Worcester, UK: International Person Centred Values Practice Network for Dementia Care.

Chappel, N.L., & Cooke, H.A. 2012. Quality of life and therapeutic environments in age related disabilities: Aging and quality of life. In *International Encyclopaedia of Rehabilitation*, edited by Stone, J.H., & Blouin, M. Available at http://cirrie.buffalo.edu/encyclopedia/.

Cunningham, C., Marshall, M., & McManus, M. 2008. *Design for Dementia Audit Tool*. Stirling, UK: University of Stirling.

Davis, S., Byers, S., & Nay, R. 2009. Guiding design of dementia friendly environments in dementia care settings. *Dementia*, 8 (2): 185–103.

Dementia Action Alliance. 2015. National Dementia Declaration for England: A Call to Action. http://www.dementiaaction.org.uk/national_alliance/downloads.

Department of Health. 2009. *Living Well with Dementia: A National Dementia Strategy.* London: Department of Health.

Department of Health. 2011. *No Health without Mental Health: A Cross-Government Mental Health Outcomes Strategy for People of All Ages.* London: Department of Health.

Department of Health. 2012. *Prime Minister's Challenge on Dementia—Delivering Major Improvements in Dementia Care and Research by 2015.* London: Department of Health.

Department of Health. 2014. *Closing the Gap: Priorities for Essential Change in Mental Health.* London: Department of Health.

Department of Health. 2015a. *Health Building Note 08-02: Dementia Friendly Health and Social Care Environments.* London: Department of Health.

Department of Health. 2015b. *Prime Minister's Challenge on Dementia 2020.* London: Department of Health.

Dutton, R. 2009. *'Extra Care' Housing and People with Dementia.* London: Housing and Dementia Research Consortium.

Evans, S., Vallelly, S., & Croucher, K. 2014. The role of specialist housing in supporting people with dementia. In *Excellence in Dementia Care*, 2nd edition, edited by Downs, M., & Bowers, B., 331–342. Maidenhead, England: Open University Press.

Ellerby, M. 2013. Schizophrenia, Maslow's hierarchy and compassion-focused therapy. *Schizophrenia Bulletin Advance Access.* doi:10.1093/schbul/sbt119.

Equality Act. (2010). legislation.gov.uk. http://www.legislation.gov.uk/ukpga/2010/15/contents

Goldstein, J.L., & Godemont, M.L. 2003. The legends and lessons of Geel, Belgium: A 1500 year old legend, a 21st century model. *Community Mental Health Journal*, 39(5): 441–458.

Joseph Rowntree Foundation. 2014. Dementia Without Walls Programme Activity and Progress. http://www.jrf.org.uk/topic/dementia-without-walls.

Kitwood, T. 1997. *Dementia Reconsidered.* Maidenhead, UK: Open University Press.

Lawton, M.P. 1977. The impact of the environment on aging and behaviour. In *Handbook of the Psychology of Aging*, edited by Birren, J.E., & Schaie, K.W., 276–301. New York: Van Nostrand.

Lawton, M.P., & Nahemow, L. 1973. Ecology and the aging process. In *The Psychology of Adult Development and Aging*, edited by Eisdorfer, C., & Lawton, M.P., 619–674. Washington, DC: American Psychological Association.

Loveday, B., Kitwood, T., & Bowe, B. 1998. *Improving Dementia Care: A Resource for Training and Professional Development.* London: Hawker.

MacDonald, R.G. 2014. The city as a laboratory of shadows: Exposing secret histories while thinking of the future. *Architecture, Media, Politics, Society*, 4(1): 1–15.

Marshall, M. 2001. Environment: How it helps to see dementia as a disability. *Journal of Dementia Care*, 6(1): 15–17.

Mental Capacity Act of 2005. 2005. http://www.legislation.gov.uk/ukpga/2005/9/contents.

MI Liverpool. 2013. MI Smarthouse. http://www.moreindependent.co.uk/life-enhancements/smarthouse/.

National Institute for Health and Clinical Excellence/Social Care Institute for Excellence Guidance. 2006. *Dementia: Supporting People with Dementia and Their Carers in Health and Social Care.* London: NICE/SCIE.

National Institute for Health and Clinical Excellence/Social Care Institute for Excellence Guidance. 2007. *DEMENTIA: The NICE/SCIE Guideline in Supporting People with Dementia and Their Carers in Health and Social Care.* Social Care Institute for Excellence and National Institute for Health and Clinical Excellence. Leicester, UK: British Psychological Society.

NHS England. 2014. *Commissioning for Quality and Innovation (CQUIN) 2014/15 Guidance*. London: NHS Commissioning Board.

Petch, A. 2014. Extending the Housing Options for Older People: Focus on Extra Care. http://www.iriss.org.uk/resources/extending-housing-options-older-people-focus-extra-care.

Wahl, H.W., Iwarsson, I., & Oswald, F. 2012. Aging well and the environment: Toward an integrative model and research agenda for the future. *The Gerontologist*, 52(3): 306–316.

World Health Organisation. 2007. *ICD 10 Version 2007*. Geneva, Switzerland: World Health Organisation.

Woods, L., Smith, G., Pendleton, J., & Parker, D. 2013. *Innovate Dementia Baseline Report: Shaping the Future for People Living with Dementia*. Liverpool, UK: Liverpool John Moores University.

Zeisel, J., Silversteen, N.M., Hyde, J., Levkoff, S., Powell Lawton, M., & Holmes, W. 2003. Environmental correlates to behavioral health outcomes in Alzheimer's special care units. *The Gerontologist*, 43(5): 697–711.

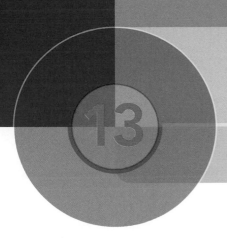

End of life care

SUSAN ASHTON

AIM

- To explore the end of life within a dementia care context

OBJECTIVES

- Introduce and identify the appropriateness of a palliative care approach for people with advanced dementia
- Recognise the role of the family carers when planning end of life care for people with dementia and understand the role of advance care planning and its role in supporting palliative care priorities
- Identify the potential end of life care needs when caring for people with dementia, including the management of symptoms and the potential ethical issues

OVERVIEW

Palliative care is a philosophy of care for the dying person and in developed countries had originally focused on the needs of people with cancer (Parker & Froggatt, 2011). Palliative care according to the World Health Organisation (WHO, 2002: 1) 'improves the quality of life of patients and families who face life-threatening illness, by providing pain and symptom relief, spiritual and psychosocial support from diagnosis to the end of life and bereavement' (WHO, 2002, 2011).

Dame Cicely Saunders was the founder of St Christopher's Hospice in 1967 and taught the concepts of 'total pain' which addresses the issues of physical, mental, social and spiritual elements to pain and distress and is well established in palliative care (WHO, 2011;

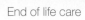

Milligan & Potts, 2009). Since 1967, the modern hospice movement and palliative care have gathered momentum and the numbers of specialist palliative care services, physicians and nurses have continually increased across the United Kingdom and Europe (WHO, 2011; Baldwin, 2011; European Association for Palliative Care [EAPC], 2007).

In recent years it has been recognised that dementia should also incorporate a palliative care approach from diagnosis until death. The National Institute for Health and Clinical Excellence (NICE) (2006) produced guidelines suggesting that regardless of where the person dies, it is important to consider the physical, psychological, social and spiritual needs of the person with dementia and the person's family. However the National Council for Palliative Care (NCPC) recognises there are challenges to providing palliative and end of life care for people with dementia. These include the unpredictable disease trajectory of dementia; the need for appropriate education and training for all health and social care professionals; and the need for further resources and access to specialist palliative care professionals (NCPC, 2010, 2009a, 2009b).

Most people with dementia also have at least one other comorbidity and often present with complex physical and psychological needs, particularly in the later stage of the disease (Sampson et al., 2008). In the advanced stage of the disease, a person with dementia is at a higher risk for hospitalisation due to an increased susceptibility to recurrent urinary tract infections as bladder function diminishes, pneumonia caused by aspiration as the swallowing mechanism declines and hip fracture as a result of falling due to the diminishing capacity of brain function (Lindstrom et al., 2011a).

One of the emerging major problems for clinicians is deciding when someone with dementia may be entering the 'dying phase'. In recognition of this, prognostic indicator guidance has been developed in the United Kingdom in an attempt to assist generalist practitioners to identify earlier when people with life-limiting diseases enter the end stage (Gold Standards Framework [GSF], 2011; Thomas, 2010a, 2010b; DH, 2008). The following are three triggers that suggest that patients are nearing the end of life:

1. The surprise question: 'Would you be surprised if this patient were to die in the next few months/weeks/days'?
2. General indicators of decline: deterioration, increasing need or choice for no further active care.
3. Specific clinical indicators related to certain conditions.

To frame our learning journey through the chapter/let us consider the following scenario:

Jean is 69 years old and is diagnosed with Alzheimer's disease. She was admitted to the Beeches Nursing Home six months ago following deterioration in her physical and mental condition. Prior to this admission Jean lived with her husband Geoff. They have four children who are married and live away from home. Jean has continued to deteriorate slowly over the last nine months. Following a review of her nursing needs it has been decided that she will be transferred to the nursing care unit of the nursing home. The nursing care unit is able to meet the needs of frail residents with an advanced stage of dementia and to plan for their end of life care needs.

We return to Jean in each section of this chapter, applying our learning as we progress through the chapter.

END OF LIFE DECISIONS

End of life decisions for people with advanced dementia are reported as often difficult for families as they attempt to make appropriate and justified decisions within the context of the person's life story (person centred). Anticipatory grief and isolation has been identified and acknowledged due to the often lengthy disease trajectory of dementia and the difficulties associated with maintaining relationships as a result of deteriorating communication and memory loss (Lindstrom et al., 2011b). Misunderstandings due to knowledge deficits and unresolved grief can have an impact on care-planning outcomes, and it is essential that this is acknowledged by nursing and other care setting staff. Open and honest conversations in which the family carers can express their anxieties and concerns should be facilitated and actively encouraged. Let us return to the chapter scenario:

Jean has now been a resident in the nursing care unit for 6 weeks. Following a case review with the general practitioner (GP) and nursing team and using the GSF Prognostic Indicators it was agreed that Jean is likely to continue to deteriorate and that palliative care should now be actively in place to meet her ongoing care needs. Jean's death was not imminent at this stage but the team agreed she was expected to deteriorate over the next few months. It was also agreed that an advance care planning (ACP) meeting should be held with Geoff, who has lasting power of attorney, to prepare and discuss Jean's potential end of life care needs.

The World Health Organisation (WHO, 2011: 11) describes ACP as a 'discussion about preferences of future care between an individual and a care provider in anticipation of future deterioration'. The Department of Health (DH, 2007: 4) clarified ACP as '… a process of discussion between an individual and their care providers irrespective of discipline … which takes place in the context of an anticipated deterioration in the individual's condition in the future with an attendant loss of capacity to make decisions and/or ability to communicate wishes to others'.

The expectation is that ACP will develop into a shared decision-making process, initiated earlier in the disease so an ongoing discussion can be facilitated to promote patient choice as much as possible. This is particularly relevant for people with dementia who may be several months or years into the disease before a confirmed diagnosis is made. In the absence of an ACP completed by the person with dementia, the family caregiver may be called on to identify and support the care choices made on the person's behalf and should be given the same level of support and consideration. It should be anticipated that some people with dementia and their family members might find these discussions distressing so care should be taken as to when and how these are facilitated.

The point at which an ACP becomes imperative to the person with dementia often involves recognition of the terminal phase of the disease, which can be problematic for health professionals. Difficult decisions often relate to the continuation or withdrawal of medical treatment and interventions such as medication, feeding tubes, treatment for newly diagnosed conditions and the appropriateness of other investigations, such as blood tests, which may not be appropriate to the dying person. The ACP process could also include personal care issues such as the preferred place of death and any funeral choices the person may have expressed.

Advance care planning has a role to play in ensuring quality terminal care but does not guarantee it (Downs, 2011). Ideally ACP should be undertaken with people with dementia before they become incapacitated. Under the terms of the Mental Capacity Act (MCA; DH, 2005), formalised outcomes of the ACP might include one of the following (Barber, Brown, & Martin, 2012; DH, 2010): advance statements to inform subsequent best interests decisions; advance decisions to refuse treatments, with these decisions legally binding if valid and applicable to the circumstances in hand; and appointment of lasting power of attorney (health and welfare or property and affairs). Less formally, the person may wish to name someone they wish to be consulted if they lose mental capacity. This is only relevant to the care and treatment of a person once the person has lost mental capacity to make decisions about any future care and treatment options. This is a legal document. It allows someone to act as an 'attorney' to make decisions on behalf of someone when that person lacks the mental capacity to do so in relation to financial affairs or personal welfare. A lasting power of attorney cannot be used until it is registered with the Office of the Public Guardian (Barber, Brown, & Martin, 2012; HM Government, 2012).

There is currently limited evidence that ACP could potentially contribute to timely palliative care interventions (van der Steen, 2010). However it is accepted that knowledge about a person's preferences for end of life care can be beneficial when planning future care (Hughes et al., 2007; Hertogh, 2006). Due to the sensitive nature of ACP discussions this can cause distress if not facilitated by appropriately trained staff (DH, 2010). Good quality and truthful discussions are required to avoid misunderstandings, complaints and unnecessary distress when difficult decisions have to be made.

Returning to the scenario:

Geoff had an initial meeting with Julie, the matron, to discuss Jean's frail condition and introduce the ACP document. Geoff was initially upset and distressed at having to think about his wife's end of life care. Julie was sensitive to Geoff's needs and gave him the document to discuss with his sons and daughters and think about what Jean would want at the end of her life. When Geoff was ready, Julie would then have a followup meeting to discuss the ACP. Why is it important to ascertain Geoff's readiness to discuss the ACP?

A staged introduction is preferred for some family carers who have difficulty accepting ACP and the terminal characteristics of the disease. It must be acknowledged that family carers have experienced different practices from professional care staff during their role as carer and this may add to misunderstandings and anxieties about what are acceptable or unacceptable care practices.

Geoff decided that he would not discuss the ACP with his family as he felt this was his decision. He did not want to upset his children and cause them anxieties about being involved in end of life care decisions. Julie arranged a meeting and identified some of the nursing and medical needs that sometimes arise with people who are in the final stage of dementia. These include hospitalisation, artificial nutrition, pain relief, deciding place of death, spiritual needs and comfort care. Julie also included personal issues that may be important to Jean such as favourite music, flowers and visiting arrangements (e.g. grandchildren present). Despite Geoff's distress he welcomed the opportunity to find out more about what would happen as the disease progressed and to talk about Jean's life and what wishes she had expressed to him before and during her illness. Geoff did not want Jean to die in hospital, he did not feel she would want to be artificially fed, and he wanted to make sure she was as comfortable as possible.

END OF LIFE CARE

The notion of dying resulting in a 'good death' plays an important role in palliative care but dying is a complex phenomenon that involves physical, emotional, psychological and social complexities (Woods, 2007). Concepts of a good death are often described using the terms comfort, peaceful, pain free, dignified, autonomous, and free from distress and suffering (Higgins, 2010; Costello, 2004). Bad deaths are associated with poor management, stress, uncontrolled pain and other bodily disintegration, poor communication, organisational and structural constraints (rules and inflexible routines) and indifference by nursing staff and doctors. Kellehear (2011: 25) states that 'the ultimate answer [to a good death] cannot be divorced from the question of what societies believe constitutes a good death [and] what it means to die well'.

The diagnosis of dying for someone with dementia is difficult due to a gradual spiral of decline, especially in the advanced stages of the disease. If the prognosis is unclear to health professionals, this may delay the discussions of dying with the person with dementia (if possible) and with the person's family (Parker & Froggatt, 2011). In the advanced stages of the disease communication abilities decline, and often health professionals and family carers need to discuss the implications of initiating a palliative care approach and continuing or withdrawing some treatment options (Hertogh, 2006). Recognising dying may include:

- Deterioration day by day because of the underlying condition
- Reduced cognition, with the individual drowsy or comatose
- Bed-bound existence or sleeping in bed most or all of the time
- Little food or fluid intake and eventual difficulty taking oral medication
- Peripheral cyanosis or coldness
- Altered breathing pattern

In light of this let us consider Jean's case:

Jean's condition deteriorated slowly over the next eight weeks. She was now in bed all day and she had difficulty taking oral fluids and nutrition. Her medication had been reviewed by the GP twice over the last eight weeks and Jean was now taking only analgesic medication as required. Her pain needs were being assessed using an observational pain assessment tool (Abbey Pain Scale). Jean was still able to take sips of water and this was being monitored by the nursing team. The GP and the nursing team agreed that Jean was now at the end of life but would be still monitored closely for any sign of improvement. Geoff was asked to review the ACP and discuss any issues or concerns he may have.

Moving towards a consensus between all those involved in the care of the person with dementia may allow for a palliative approach to be developed earlier in the person's disease trajectory. However it is important to consider any other reasons for the person's physical deterioration, including reversible causes (e.g. infection, oversedation, dehydration and renal failure).

The use of prognostic indicators and care pathways may provide opportunities to guide professionals on when to initiate and deliver palliative care to people with advanced dementia. It is important to involve all professionals involved in the care of the person with dementia to obtain a team perspective on the diagnosis of dying. Discuss the change in the person's condition with the patient if possible or the family and make sure all questions are answered accurately and honestly.

It is difficult to record what constitutes a good death for people with dementia as little is known about the dying phase. However certain key issues are reported, including being 'pain free', 'dying in preferred place', 'comfort care', and the 'avoidance of inappropriate investigations and interventions'. Communication difficulties and lack of responsiveness in the later stages of the disease may be interpreted by health and social care professionals to mean that spiritual, religious and cultural needs are no longer applicable. This approach would be insensitive and inappropriate.

Issues of personhood and the value of life of the person with dementia, first described by Kitwood (1997), have been identified as important yet challenging, especially as individuals move towards the advanced stage of their disease (Killick, 2006; MacKinley, 2006). Communication and the ability to engage in everyday interests and activities are often at the core of relationships which give life meaning. Spirituality is often associated with religious beliefs, rituals and practice (Power, 2006), and a person with advanced dementia may not be in a position to fully participate due to their cognitive impairment and communication loss. However it is increasingly acknowledged that religious beliefs and practices may be only one dimension of spiritual care (MacKinley, 2006; Killick, 2006). It is important to respect the person's differences and work closely with the person's family to ensure all their care needs are addressed.

SYMPTOM MANAGEMENT

The Leadership Alliance for the Care of Dying People (2014) has produced a report and recommendations following a review of how end of life care was being interpreted and delivered by health-care professionals. The review found variations in care for dying people which could and sometimes did result in poor standards of care. The report emphasises the priorities of care that are required when it is thought a person is dying.

The individualised plan of care should consider the following:

- Stopping any unnecessary treatments and medications.
- Reconsidering route of appropriate medications.
- Anticipating prescribing which may be required as the person with dementia approaches the end of their life. Medications might include cyclizine, diamorphine, hyoscine hydrobromide and midazolam.
- Controlling physical symptoms.
- Having realistic goals (e.g. do not attempt resuscitation[DNAR]).
- Preparing the environment of dying. Has the person completed an ACP indicating any preferences?
- Handing over forms to out-of-hours care. This is essential to ensure continuity of care out of hours if the person is in a nursing home or their own home.

A multiprofessional team approach should always be adopted when planning care for people who are at the end of life regardless of the disease. This must include access to specialist palliative care teams and should also include the family carers in all discussions. The care plan must be reviewed every 4 hours at a minimum to ensure that appropriate care is being delivered. Daily medical review and re-evaluation is also necessary to ensure the plan of care is meeting the needs of the dying person and that the confirmation of the dying phase is still appropriate. Members of the multiprofessional team who could be involved in the care of the dying person could include the following:

- Palliative care team
- Medical staff
- Speech and language therapist
- Advanced nurse practitioners
- Tissue viability nurse
- Pharmacist
- Dietician
- Chaplains if requested

The person with dementia may not be able to articulate that he or she has pain but may present with other behaviours, such as agitation, which may be more difficult to interpret and explain. Pain observation tools or charts can be useful for assisting the nurse to recognise pain in people who are unable to communicate. The Abbey Pain Scale is a 1-minute numerical observation tool (Abbey et al., 2004). PAINAD (Pain Assessment in Advanced Dementia) is another valuable pain observation tool that can be used to assist the nurse in identifying pain and discomfort in the person with dementia at the end of life (Warden, Hurley, & Volicer, 2003). The focus of these pain observation tools is to identify behaviour and other factors (e.g. pressure sores) which may contribute to the person being in pain if he or she cannot communicate needs to nursing and care staff. The person may also not present with psychological distress that can be observed visually, particularly in the last few months or weeks as communication diminishes. However psychological distress cannot be ignored just because the person is unable to articulate this. Nursing and care staff should ensure the care they deliver is compassionate and dignified.

Returning to the scenario:

Jean's status was reviewed by the GP and palliative care nurse and it was agreed that the recommended end of life care medication be prescribed in anticipation of her needs. This included diamorphine, midazolam and hyoscine hydrobromide. Over the next 72 hours, Jean's condition deteriorated, but she appeared comfortable and not distressed, so the medication was not administered. Geoff was with Jean when she died. Jean died with her favourite music playing and her family (including her grandchildren) around her in the nursing home.

THE ETHICAL CONTEXT

If a diagnosis of dying is difficult for health professionals, then this will impact on the care and treatment plans to which the person may be exposed. Ethical care does not include subjecting the person to any distressing investigations and treatments which may be of questionable benefit. In the advanced stages of the disease there are ethical issues that can impact on the quality of care and experience of dying. Artificial hydration and nutrition, pain relief and medication management are examples of the ethical dilemmas that health professionals may encounter (Parsons et al., 2010; Kumar & Kuriakose, 2013). Care and treatment should be judged on the amount of discomfort related to it and if this is what the person would have wanted had they been able to express an opinion. Ethical issues might include:

- Withdrawal of aggressive or active treatment. This could include the need for invasive investigations, X-rays, blood tests, investigation of new symptoms not related to the dementia (e.g. cancer symptoms).

- Withdrawal of previous medication. People with dementia often have multiple medications which may be prescribed as a result of behaviour management in the later stages or as a result of other comorbidities (e.g. cardiovascular disorders, diabetes).
- Hydration and nutrition. People in the advanced stage of disease often have difficulty swallowing. Nasogastric tubes/percutaneous endoscopic gastrostomy feeding tubes are often poorly tolerated and may not increase survival or may worsen aspiration. Short-term nonoral hydration may be managed with subcutaneous hydration.
- Pain relief (double effect). Pain relief is beneficial to the dying person if the person has been assessed as being in pain. A potential consequence of strong analgesia or narcotic pain relief may have the effect of shortening the life expectancy of the person, known as the 'double effect'.
- When and if to continue with pressure area care in the later stages, particularly if the person becomes distressed on movement.
- Environment of care. Patients are often at risk of hospitalisation if community support services are inadequate or not in place.
- Moral or religious conflict. Relatives may have unrealistic expectations of treatment or may have difficulties accepting their loved one is dying.
- Time to care. Staffing shortages and competing demands in the caring environment may make it challenging to give the dying person sufficient time to care for their needs.

It is important to recognise the ongoing needs of the person as well as the needs of the family members. Care after death may need to include any cultural or religious needs, so prompt certification may be required. Family members may require bereavement support so having access to this information may be useful.

CHAPTER SUMMARY

No two people with dementia are the same and this is also applicable at the end of life.

Due to the often gradual decline, which may be over several years, it is frequently difficult for clinicians to diagnose when the person has entered the dying phase.

Clinical guidelines, prognostic indicators and observational pain management tools can be useful when planning palliative and comfort care.

An individualised assessment and care plan are essential, which should take account of any previous ACP discussions.

Symptom management should be reviewed frequently and based on a multiprofessional approach to ensure the person's needs are met at the end of life. This should include examination of food and drink, symptom control and psychological, social and spiritual support which is agreed, coordinated and delivered with compassion and dignity.

REFLECTION ON LEARNING

1. What is palliative care?
2. What role can an ACP have when planning palliative care for someone with dementia?
3. What information do you think should be included in an ACP?
4. What support should be offered to the patient and family when undertaking ACP discussions?

5. What presenting indicators might alert you that your patient is now in need of a palliative care approach?

6. What does the Leadership Alliance suggest should be included in a plan of care for a person who is dying?

7. Why might pain observational tools be useful when assessing the needs of the person with advanced dementia?

8. What ethical issues may need to be considered when caring for a person with dementia who is at the end of life?

9. Why is it important to review the condition of the person with dementia regularly even though the person may be considered at the end of life?

10. What is a good death?

REFERENCES

Abbey, J., Piller, N., DeBellis, A., Esterman, A., Parker, D., Giles, L., & Lawcay, B. 2004. The Abbey Pain Scale: A 1 minute numerical indicator for people with end-stage dementia. *International Journal of Palliative Nursing*, 10(1): 6–13.

Baldwin, M.A. 2011. Hospice movement and evolution of palliative care. In *Key Concepts in Palliative Care*, edited by Baldwin, M.A., & Woodhouse, J., 92–96. London: Sage.

Barber, P., Brown, R., & Martin, D. 2012. *Mental Health Law in England and Wales. A Guide for Mental Health Professionals*, 2nd edition. London: Sage.

Costello, J. 2004. *Nursing the Dying Patient. Caring in Different Contexts*. Basingstoke, UK: Palgrave Macmillan.

Department of Health. 2005. *Mental Capacity Act*. London: HMSO.

Department of Health. 2007. *Advance Care Planning. A Guide for Health and Social Care Staff*. London: Department of Health.

Department of Health. 2008. *End of Life Care Strategy—Promoting High Quality Care for Adults at the End of Life*. London: Department of Health.

Department of Health. 2010. *Quality Outcomes for People with Dementia: Building on the Work of the National Dementia Strategy*. London: Department of Health.

Downs, M. 2011. End of Life care for older people with dementia: Priorities for research and service development. In *Living with Ageing and Dying: Palliative and End of Life Care for Older People*, edited by Gott, M., & Ingleton, C. Oxford, UK: Oxford University Press.

European Association of Palliative Care. 2012. White Paper on Dementia. http://www.eapcnet.eu/Themes/Clinicalcare/EAPCWhitepaperondementia.aspx.

Gold Standards Framework. 2011. *The Gold Standards Framework Prognostic Indicator Guidance*, 4th edition. http://www.goldstandardsframework.org.uk/.

Hertogh, C.M.P.M. 2006. Advance care planning and the relevance of a palliative care approach in dementia. *Age and Ageing*, 35(6): 553–555.

Higgins, D. 2010. Care of the dying patient. A guide for nurses. In *Care of the Dying and Deceased Patient. A Practical Guide for Nurses*, edited by Jevon, P., 1–36. Chichester, UK: Wiley-Blackwell.

HM Government. 2012. Lasting Power of Attorney. https://www.gov.uk/power-of-attorney/overview.

Hughes, J.C., Jolley, D., Jordon, A., & Sampson, E.L. 2007. Palliative care in dementia: Issues and evidence. *Advances in Psychiatric Treatment*, 13: 251–260.

Kellehear, A. 2011. The care of older people at the end of life: A critical perspective. In *Living with Ageing and Dying: Palliative and End of Life Care for Older People*, edited by Gott, M., & Ingleton, C. Oxford, UK: Oxford University Press.

Killick, J. 2006. Helping the flame to stay bright: Celebrating the spiritual in dementia. *Journal of Religion, Spirituality and Aging*, 18(2): 73–78.

Kitwood, T. 1997. *Dementia Reconsidered*. Buckingham, UK: Open University Press.

Leadership Alliance for the Care of Dying People. 2014. One Chance to Get it Right. http://www.gov.uk/government/publications/liverpool-care-pathway-review-response-to-recommendations.

Lindstrom, K.B., Bosch, R., Cohen, R.M., Fredericks, P., Hall, G.R., Harrington, P., Hollawell, D., et al. 2011a. The continuum of care. In *Palliative Care for Advanced Alzheimer's and Dementia. Guidelines and Standards for Evidence Based Care*, edited by Martin, G.A., & Sabbagh, M.N., 11–24. New York: Springer.

Lindstrom, K.B., Bosch, R., Cohen, R.M., Fredericks, P., Hall, G.R., Harrington, P., Hollawell, D., et al. 2011b. The continuum of grief. In *Palliative Care for Advanced Alzheimer's and Dementia. Guidelines and Standards for Evidence Based Care*, edited by Martin, G.A., & Sabbagh, M.N., 259–270. New York: Springer.

MacKinley, E. 2006. Spiritual care: Recognizing spiritual needs of older adults. *Journal of Religion, Spirituality and Aging*, 18(2): 59–71.

Milligin, S., & Potts, S. 2009. The history of palliative care. In *Palliative Nursing Across the Spectrum of Care*, edited by Stevens, E., Jackson, S., & Milligan, S., 5–16. Chichester, UK: Wiley Blackwell.

National Council for Palliative Care. 2009a. *Out of the Shadows: End of Life Care for People with Dementia*. London: National Council for Palliative Care.

National Council for Palliative Care. 2009b. *The Power of Partnership: Palliative Care in Dementia*. London: National Council for Palliative Care.

National Council for Palliative Care. 2010. *End of Life Quality Markers for Dementia: Joint Guide to Using Quality Markers to Join Up Dementia and End of Life Strategies*. London: National Council for Palliative Care.

Parker, D., & Froggatt, K. 2011. Palliative care with older people. In *Evidence Informed Nursing with Older People*, edited by Tolson, D., Booth, J., & Schofield, I. Chichester, UK: Wiley-Blackwell.

Sampson, E.L., Thune-Boyle, I., Kukkastenvehmas, R., Jones, L., Tookman, A., King, M., & Blanchard, M.R. 2008. Palliative care in advanced dementia: A mixed methods approach for the development of a complex intervention. *BMC Palliative Care*, 7(8). doi:10.1186/1472-684X-7-8.

Thomas, K. 2010a. Prognostic Indicator Guidance to assist generalist clinicians with early identification of people approaching the end stage of their disease process. *End of Life Care*, 4(1). http://endoflifejournal.stchristophers.org.uk/gold-standards-framework/the-gsf-prognostic-indicator-guidance.

Thomas, K. 2010b. Using prognostic indicator guidance to plan care for final stages of life. *Primary Health Care*, 20(6): 25–28.

Van der Steen, J.T. 2010. Dying with dementia: What we know after more than a decade of research. *Journal of Alzheimer's Disease*, 22: 37–55.

Warden, V., Hurley, A.C., & Volicer, L. 2003. Development and psychometric evaluation of the Pain Assessment in Advanced Dementia (PAINAD) scale. *Journal of the American Medical Directors Association*, 4(1): 9–15.

Woods, S. 2007. *Death's Dominion. Ethics at the End of Life.* Berkshire, UK: Open University Press.

World Health Organisation. 2002. WHO definition of palliative care. *http://who.int/cancer/palliative/definition*.

World Health Organisation. 2011. *Palliative Care for Older People: Better Practices.* Rome: WHO.

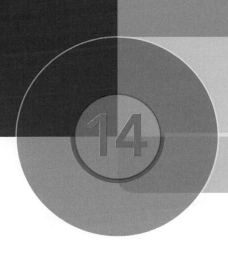

Research

DAZ GREENOP AND GRAHAME SMITH

AIM

- To explore how research can enable people living with dementia to live well

OBJECTIVES

- Identify the different types of research, including scientific, naturalistic, participatory, and pragmatic approaches
- Consider how dementia-related research can be applied to practice
- Reflect on the importance of involving people living with dementia in the research process

OVERVIEW

Historically, funding for dementia research has been significantly lower than for other long-term conditions. While dementia accounts for 50% of the combined health-care costs of cancer, coronary heart disease and stroke, it receives only a fraction of the combined research funding for these conditions (Alzheimer's Research Trust, 2010). There is, however, reason to believe that this inequity is finally being addressed, with annual research expenditure doubling to £60 million between the Prime Minister's *first* 'challenge on dementia' in 2012 and his *second* in 2015. Funding is set to double again by 2025 (Department of Health, 2015).

The infrastructure is changing too with the establishment of the Dementia Research Institute in England and stronger partnerships between industry, academia, research charities, NHS and the private sector. Perhaps most importantly there needs to be an increase of people with dementia participating in research, and the government has set a target of 25% of people diagnosed with dementia becoming registered on Join Dementia Research and 10% participating in research, up from the current baseline of 4.5% (Department of Health, 2015). Through these initiatives and others the British government hopes to make the UK 'the best place for dementia research through a partnership between patients, researchers, funders and society' (Department of Health, 2015 p. 46).

The challenge ahead is great and getting greater every day as the population of people with dementia is set to more than double by 2050 (Alzheimer's Society, 2007; Woods et al., 2013) creating a social and economic 'burden' that could further prejudice public attitudes and diminish the quality of care and support provided (Woods et al., 2013). Research has had a central role in enabling people with dementia to live long lives and it now has a responsibility to ensure they live well (Department of Health, 2009). As highlighted in the Alzheimer's Society (2012) report people living with dementia clearly view research within this area as a priority:

> Eighty-three per cent of respondents said that research into improving care for people now was important; 83% said that research into the cause was important and 87% said that research into the cure was important. 82% of respondents also felt that there should be more funding for dementia research. (Alzheimer's Society, 2012: Executive Summary)

This chapter explores four common research approaches, with examples, that can be utilised by health and social care professionals to help people with dementia live well. While these four approaches are very different they are not necessarily contradictory but may be used to develop a multidimensional, evidence-based framework that can transform practice. With this in mind, brief examples of relevant research are presented in the section on research types. This will encourage the reader to critically question narrow 'quantocentric' thinking. We then analyse how different approaches could be applied to practice. Lastly, but just as important, we consider how people with dementia can be engaged meaningfully within the research process.

TYPES OF RESEARCH

Practitioners do not exclusively use one source of knowledge but draw on many interconnecting streams of information, understanding and evidence which, consciously and unconsciously, coalesce in their everyday decision-making (Greenhalgh & Wieringa, 2011; Smith, 2014). Research is therefore just one of many intellectual resources alongside, for example, traditional and routine-based knowledge and experience-based knowledge. Importantly, these different sources of knowledge constantly interact with each other, straddling and challenging the supposed research-practice divide (Greenhalgh & Wieringa, 2011). Research may, for example, suggest that practitioners should change practice in a certain way but experience may modify this change, which then becomes the norm or traditional practice (Finfgeld-Connett, 2008; Smith, 2012). Conversely, innovations in practice may challenge old assumptions and inspire new hypotheses for researchers to investigate further. Either way, research is a systematic way of gaining knowledge so that, whether working from the 'top down' or 'bottom up', what is already known is added to, rejected or confirmed (Greenhalgh & Wieringa, 2011).

Historically health and social care professionals have mostly utilised top-down research methods. Generally these have been 'scientific' and quantitative in nature, but practitioners are increasingly interested in more 'naturalistic' qualitative approaches (Greenhalgh & Wieringa, 2011; Smith, 2014). Scientific methods focus on objectively measuring cause and effect while naturalistic approaches focus on subjectively evaluating meaning and experience. Either way these approaches remain researcher led and provide little opportunity for participants to contribute meaningfully to the research agenda. To address this, some researchers and practitioners within health and social care have recently been adopting more pragmatic problem-solving techniques and participatory methods (Johnson et al., 2007). Both are focussed on change and involve bottom-up thinking; they are more typically user led in relation to the design and dissemination of research.

Research may be utilised *retrospectively* to justify, or challenge, past actions or it may be utilised *prospectively* to inform future actions. The latter in particular is commonly referred to as evidence-based practice (EBP), which Sackett et al. (1996 p.71) describe as '... the conscientious, explicit and judicious application of current best evidence in making decisions'. EBP enables practitioners to provide a high standard of care with improved outcomes for people with dementia. Practitioners have a tendency to generalise quantocentric EBP as a shorthand way of talking about research but it is important to recognise that this only provides one perspective which can often be a limited way of understanding evidence. A better understanding can be engendered through what has been described as multidimensional EBP, which Petr and Walter (2009, p. 231) suggest 'redefines best practices by incorporating consumer, professional and quantitative research in the best practices inquiry, thus empowering those doing the work and receiving the services'. Multidimensional EBP therefore acknowledges multiple sources of evidence which are context dependent so practitioners need to be able to critically evaluate it to justify its use in a particular setting.

Scientific research approaches take different forms but all assume that knowledge is factual and arises from experiment and observation. Theory is grounded in the certainty of sense experience or rational argument with the aim of achieving generalisability. Quantitative methods such as surveys, documentary evidence, and randomised controlled trials are used to establish what works. Together these dominate dementia research but it is important to recognise that this is a decontextualised and ideal type of evidence that may not always be practicable or ethical (e.g. if it involves withholding necessary medical treatment from control groups). It is also important to note that this type of evidence is provisional and continually being updated, so on this basis practitioners need to ensure they also are regularly updated about any advances. This should include checking any relevant clinical guidelines which are shaped by EBP as the evidence changes. Evidence-based practice has a number of steps which start with asking a clinical question, such as, What is the best nursing intervention for this condition? The practitioner will then move on to

- Identify the relevant literature that helps address the question
- Critically assess the evidence, asking whether it is reliable or valid
- Apply the chosen evidence
- Evaluate the application of the evidence

Let us consider these points in relation to the following example:

Crooks et al. (2008) examined whether social networks had a protective association with incidence of dementia among elderly women. The researchers prospectively studied 2,249 members of a health maintenance organisation who were 78 years or older, were classified as free of dementia in 2001, and had completed at least one follow-up interview in 2002 through 2005. They used a number of validated research tools to collect data by telephone on cognitive status and social networks. The researchers identified 268 cases of dementia during follow-up and observed that compared with women with smaller social networks, the adjusted hazard ratio for incident dementia in women with larger social networks was 0.74 (95% confidence interval = 0.57, 0.97). The researchers therefore concluded that larger social networks have a protective influence on cognitive function among elderly women.

Naturalistic research approaches also take many forms but all assume that knowledge is personal and arises from insight and intuition. The aim of these approaches is to achieve increased (empathic) understanding rather than merely explaining behaviours in terms of causes and correlates. In-depth interviewing, focus groups, participant observation and other naturalistic methods are therefore used to explore human experience, meaning and potential. Some of the different approaches using these methods include the following:

- Phenomenology: Describing phenomena (free from preconception) through how they are perceived by research participants
- Grounded theory: Generating new theories by systematically collecting, coding, conceptualising and categorising qualitative data
- Ethnography: Documenting the culture, perspectives and practices and all symbol-meaning relations of people in their natural setting
- Narrative analysis: Exploring how people create and use stories to make sense of change in their lives
- Case study: Analysing an instance of a class of phenomena (person, group or event) holistically over time, usually relying on multiple sources of evidence

Despite their many differences, all of these approaches seek to get inside the lifeworld of the research subject by exploring the meanings of their words and actions. As in scientific inquiry, there is an ongoing debate regarding how 'pure' the knowledge generated can be but unlike scientists, qualitative researchers do not necessarily seek to eradicate 'error' (such as personal perspective and interpretation) from the data they gather but rather acknowledge errors as integral to the research process. The following example relates to an ethnographic approach:

Ericsson, Hellström and Kjellström (2011) undertook an ethnography describing how people with dementia interact with cognitively intact co-residents (including caregivers) in housing with care for the elderly in Sweden. During fieldwork they observed nine people with dementia on a total of 31 occasions during meals and other planned activities. On conclusion, the researchers expanded their field notes into a more detailed narrative. To achieve deeper understanding, semistructured interviews were then undertaken with nine contact persons who were 'highly familiar with the persons observed' (p. 525) and were able to corroborate what had been observed. Finally, a few informal interviews were undertaken with the research subjects themselves to clarify aspects of interaction that remained difficult to explain.

The researchers described and explored different interactions in their results on a 'sliding scale' of verbal and non-verbal expressions of satisfaction, disorientation or dissociation which, they argued, do not simply depend on degree of cognitive ability but on a number of contextual factors such as whether others make an effort to involve them, how others react to them and how they are treated. For example, residents with dementia seldom initiated extended interaction and quickly sank 'into their own world' unless something demanded their attention. If, however, there were people around to initiate and sustain one-to-one interaction, this promoted expressions of satisfaction. The researchers' careful analysis of verbal and non-verbal emotional expressions suggests that residents' awareness was probably greater than many of the caregivers realised and they concluded it is important always to assume that people with dementia understand their situation and the way that those around them behave toward them.

Traditional qualitative or quantitative methods may be criticised for using research participants to 'extract' data without providing time or space for them to frame, interpret or explain the meaning of their words or actions. Participatory action research (PAR) directly addresses this issue.

It is difficult to define PAR because, as Fals-Borda (1997: 111) noted, it is 'a philosophy of life as much as a method, a sentiment as much as a conviction'. Methodologically it is eclectic, using whatever tools are needed to maximise participation and achieve its goals. Unlike traditional research however participation is not a means to an end but an end in itself. One of the distinguishing features of PAR therefore is the inclusion of participants in *all* phases of the research from design to dissemination so that participation is optimised throughout the research process. Whether utilising quantitative, qualitative or mixed methods, consciousness raising and the empowerment of research participants are its goal (Eckhardt & Anastas, 2007).

PAR questions the usefulness and even possibility of pure uncontaminated and 'value-free' data (whether quantitatively or qualitatively generated) in the real world. Rather, it starts from the overt value position that some groups in society (including people with dementia) are disadvantaged, marginalised and silenced by oppressive social structures. PAR therefore seeks to privilege their role in research and encourages their active collaboration in challenging dominant discourses and 'received wisdom' throughout the research process either individually or collectively. Knowledge is therefore reconstructed from the 'bottom up', making links between personal experience, local issues and structural inequality. By building collective insights among people with dementia, PAR can deepen their sense of identity and interconnectedness and challenge the processes by which their oppression is internalised and sustained; for example:

Drawing on cognitive rehabilitation theory, Nomura et al. (2009) used PAR to develop a group activity programme for 37 community-dwelling people with dementia and education and counselling programmes for 31 family caregivers in rural Japan. The research evolved over three cycles of planning, action and reflection at individual, group, and community levels. The main focus of the first cycle was the development of an intervention to regain procedural skills through a cooking programme. The second cycle focussed on increasing interactions between family members and with other people with dementia through group activities that promoted communication. In the third cycle, culturally relevant sequential activities were undertaken. The researchers used three data sources to create a portfolio for each person with the dementia-caregiver dyad drawing on (1) a semistructured observation sheet, (2) a communication notebook for caregivers to take home and record activity and observed changes after the group activities and (3) the content of monthly phone interviews with caregivers. According to the authors, the project helped people with dementia restore lost procedural skills and regain confidence. It also illustrated the importance of interventions that target both (community-dwelling) people with dementia and their family caregivers, concluding, 'The recognition of their skills by the group members and by their families appeared to be the most powerful component of empowerment' (p. 440).

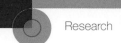

Research is often caricatured as an abstract academic activity undertaken in sterile laboratory conditions. With some justification it may be accused of having little or no relevance to everyday challenges that practitioners face as they endeavour to develop health and social care that is effective and of good quality. It is however possible to undertake *real* research pragmatically in what has been described and developed as a 'living lab' approach.

A Living Lab is a user-centric innovation milieu built on everyday practice and research, with an approach that facilitates user influence in open and distributed innovation processes engaging all relevant partners in real-life contexts, aiming to create sustainable values. (Bergvall-Kåreborn & Ståhlbröst, 2010: 191)

The challenges practitioners face in the real world can occur at both a macro level, being part of a wider service delivering care, and at a micro level, delivering direct face-to-face care. As resources become scarce or care becomes more complex the practitioner is required to develop and apply new and different solutions—in other words innovate. Pragmatic approaches such as the living lab provide a way of ensuring that innovations are both useful and usable by involving end users in the problem-solving process (Woods et al., 2013). Living labs therefore focus on harnessing the knowledge and expertise which users bring to the collaborative process to achieve shared learning (Woods et al., 2013).

At an application level living labs have the characteristics of PAR with a focus on developing 'practical knowing through a participatory process' akin to action research (Reason & Bradbury, 2001; Reason, 2003; Budweg et al., 2015). The approach emerged from an information communication technology background and may be linked rather with the philosophical pragmatism of Richard Rorty, by which ideas are valued in terms of their 'usefulness, workability, and practicality' (Johnson et al., 2007; Reason, 2003). The Innovate Dementia project is an example of this approach in action:

Innovate Dementia is a European- (Interreg IVB [area]) funded project which aims to establish living labs across northwestern Europe to test and evaluate innovative dementia care models. Bringing people with dementia (and family caregivers) together with health and social care professionals, academics and business in a 'triple helix' approach, these collaborative spaces provide platforms for all stakeholders to share knowledge, enhance expertise and improve performance.

The living labs established within the project explore and validate potential solutions to the challenge of living every day with dementia. These provide a dynamic structure and are driven by the real needs of people with dementia. To provide a sense of consistency and to ensure it was fit for purpose for the work of the project the definition for a living lab was further refined as

… a pragmatic research environment which openly engages all relevant partners with an emphasis on improving the real-life care of people with dementia through the use of economically viable and sustainable innovations. (Woods et al., 2013: 13–14)

The living lab approach of Innovate Dementia is now successfully influencing health innovation (models of assistance), new technologies (intelligent lighting) and lifestyles (nutrition and exercise) that may help prevent the development of dementia and enable people to live well with dementia. However, it is recognised within the project that the work of the living lab will only be successful if the proposed innovations reflect the real needs of people with dementia. On this basis the strength of using a living lab approach is that it creates an environment in which real needs of people with dementia are recognised and championed.

APPLYING RESEARCH TO PRACTICE

Social networks are increasingly recognised as protecting people from cognitive decline in later life (Crooks et al., 2008). However, not only the quantity of social contacts matter but also their quality (Fratiglioni et al., 2000). Unsurprisingly perhaps the majority of people with dementia describe themselves as lonely, particularly those who live in the community (Alzheimer's Society, 2013), suggesting the real possibility of many people becoming locked into a spiralling cycle of isolation and deterioration. While perhaps not inevitable the personal consequences of such a scenario for individuals with dementia are likely to be far reaching as both opportunity and capacity for meaningful interaction diminish (Shankar et al., 2013). More optimistically, what the isolation-connectedness hypothesis seems to be suggesting is that the depression, irritation, self-neglect and rapid decline often associated with dementia are potentially avoidable (Holwerda et al., 2014; Alzheimer's Society, 2013). Let us consider the following:

> Imagine you are a researcher-practitioner seeking to evaluate a group intervention aimed at reducing isolation for people with dementia living in the community. Using one or more of the four approaches outlined in this chapter think about how you could capture what difference the programme has made. What information would you need and how would you get it?

The validity of a scientific approach very much depends on researchers being able to analyse large data sets. In this particular scenario, this might be generated using validated tools to quantify the frequency of social contact along with levels of depression/irritation/self-neglect/decline experienced. It will also be necessary to compare findings with some kind of objective standard such as a control (or 'non-intervention') group or baseline (before/after intervention) measure. To make generalisations as meaningful as possible, researchers would need to maximise sample size. This might be achieved by devising brief and accessible structured questionnaires, which may be completed in person, by post, online or over the telephone.

The main problem with this approach is that it depends on self-reporting (or observations by family members) which can be unreliable. On a more philosophical note, the objectification of subjective experience inherent in such measures involves a confusion of epistemological categories and could be dismissed a priori as meaningless. Other, more practical issues include ensuring that specific variables can be isolated, measured and linked causally with social isolation/connectedness. How can we be sure which were (not) effective? Is it ethical? Should participants, for example, be randomly selected or allocated to intervention/control groups? In reality control groups are determined by circumstances rather than design. Evaluations of this kind are therefore likely to involve only one or two groups and will therefore lack generalizability—a key objective of scientific approaches.

Naturalistic approaches would focus on quality rather than quantity and would rely much more on the person with dementia's own accounts than on validated scales, etc. In particular semistructured interviews may be used to explore how a small number of participants changed (in relation to isolation-connectedness) as a result of the intervention. Interview questions might explore the impact of specific activities undertaken, while more open-ended questions might ask about what participants feel worked well and what did not. The stories of participants should be of central importance to this approach, so qualitative researchers would be interested in exploring individual journeys through the intervention, their unique social settings, what motivated them to join this particular social group, and so on. A major drawback of qualitative approaches is the small sample sizes and lack of representativeness, not only of the participants but also concerning the researcher, who is perhaps the most powerful of all voices. The danger therefore is that the narratives of participants are simply subsumed within the researcher's preferred interpretive framework. Qualitative research depends very much on the qualities of the researcher (as much as the quality of the data) and his or her ability to make the 'findings' as transparent as possible by highlighting the personal, social and structural assumptions influencing the research process.

PAR starts from an overt value position that people with dementia are disadvantaged. This approach would from the outset seek to privilege the participants' role in the research, encouraging their active collaboration throughout (from design to dissemination) either individually or through focus groups or community work. Participants would therefore not only be answering questions but also asking them, exploring for example ways in which ageist social structures can lead to the medicalization of loneliness and how these are enacted by the 'helping' professions (and researchers). PAR would seek to embed these questions into the intervention itself, allowing participants maximum control over the entire project. Successful outcomes would be evaluated in relation to consciousness raising and creating greater awareness of the oppressive structures exacerbating their *social* condition.

As with PAR, a pragmatic approach would start by engaging with people with dementia to establish the purpose of the intervention but not necessarily with an ideological commitment to consciousness raising and antioppressive practice. Researchers may also bring in other stakeholders (family carers, practitioners, community members) in a living lab to 'experiment' with possible ideas to develop the intervention (and suggest alternatives). Meetings would need to be regular and purposeful (passing through cycles of planning, action and reflection) and could, theoretically, continue ad infinitum or until the agreed outcomes of the intervention are achieved. This may be done collectively or participants could be organised into smaller action learning sets consisting of people connected to a specific individual with dementia who are capable of bringing about positive change and tailoring support for that person.

ENGAGING PEOPLE WITH DEMENTIA IN RESEARCH

Seventy-five per cent of respondents thought that it was either very or quite important to hear about research into dementia and 64% indicated that being asked to take part in dementia research was important for them. (Alzheimer's Society, 2012: Executive Summary)

Despite a growing interest in participation, the views, opinions and experiences of people with dementia are still routinely excluded from research (McKeown et al., 2010). Where they are included, their involvement can become tokenistic as the methods employed (questionnaires, interviews, focus groups, observation, etc.) are seldom adapted appropriately to make it meaningful (McLaughlin, 2010; McKeown et al., 2010). Tokenism is not an uncommon concern within the area of service user involvement within the research process:

> Too often, successful service user involvement has been identified solely in terms of whether service users have contributed to the completion of a research project. This neglects both a focus on outcomes and the types of knowledge claims being made. (McLaughlin, 2010: 1604)

This failure by researchers may even lead them to conclude that people with dementia lack the will, desire or capacity to make a substantive contribution (McLaughlin, 2010; McKeown et al., 2010). It can also lead to lost opportunities. Tanner's (2013) study which worked with people with dementia as coresearchers makes the point that lack of motivation was not an issue—quite the opposite. There was a need to help others with dementia, as one participant stated: 'If I could feel useful to someone, it would be quite something' (p. 301). Yes, managing capacity within the research process can be an ethical challenge, though the appropriate use of the Mental Capacity Act 2005 will assist the researcher in positively managing this challenge:

> One way of enhancing involvement is to adhere to the provisions of the act and its code of practice (Department for Constitutional Affairs, 2007). The act challenges the 'consent by proxy' approach, and has opened up the possibilities for people with dementia to be included in research and given a voice in a protected, transparent framework. (Murray, 2013: 20)

There has been a welcome effort by some researchers to address barriers to participation head on by using more flexible research methods such as biographies, life story, photos and other memory aids (Moos & Bjorn, 2006). This brings many potential benefits but if undertaken without the necessary skills and safeguards in place, the voices of people with dementia easily become dominated and their involvement may even cause unnecessary distress. Involving people with dementia in research should not therefore be regarded as good practice in and of itself, especially when it is emotionally demanding or risky and brings no obvious benefit (McLaughlin, 2010; Tanner, 2013).

Research is not always rewarding, and full participation is not always necessary. It is perhaps best understood as a continuum that at one end may simply involve *consulting* with people and at the other end offers them *complete control* (Hanley et al., 2004). Traditional approaches therefore still have an important role to play in dementia research alongside more innovative ones but wherever possible, they must be adapted appropriately (e.g. adjusting focus group size, exploring the type and stage of dementia, reducing duration of interviews, tailoring content, employing visual aids, etc.). If full participation is desirable, people with dementia must also be actively engaged in setting the research agenda as equal partners (Weber, 2011; McLaughlin, 2010), from beginning to end, not only answering the questions but also posing them. If research is truly inclusive, there can be a number of benefits. A study by Tanner (2013) highlights the potential benefits of engaging people with dementia as coresearchers:

> Our research indicates that older people with dementia can make a valuable contribution to research as both co-researchers and participants. Their involvement in the project gave them a sense of purpose and value, countering the feelings of powerlessness more

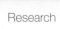

usually associated with dementia (Proctor, 2001). This form of research involvement is consistent with promoting the citizenship of people with dementia (Bartlett & O'Connor, 2007), since it recognises their capacity to exercise agency and exert influence. (Tanner, 2013: 304)

CHAPTER SUMMARY

We have considered four different approaches to research that require different levels of involvement—from mere consultation to complete control with people with dementia becoming equal partners. For involvement at any level to be meaningful, however, researchers need to be methodologically tuned to the strengths, vulnerabilities, settings and preferences of people with dementia.

The multidimensional framework presented in this chapter acknowledges and includes traditional EBP and the personal narrative of people with dementia using both top-down researcher-led and bottom-up user-led approaches. By working in this way, it becomes possible to challenge narrow thinking and gain a more holistic understanding of what it means to live well with dementia and bring about sustainable improvement.

There is an urgent need to undertake research that will enable people with dementia to live well, but to achieve this, they must be meaningfully engaged in the co-creation of knowledge and co-production of services.

REFLECTION ON LEARNING

1. What different sources of knowledge do you utilise in your daily practice?
2. What is a multidimensional evidence framework, and how can it help people with dementia to live well?
3. What is the key difference between qualitative and quantitative research?
4. How does quantitative and qualitative research differ from PAR and pragmatic research?
5. Match the following research approaches to an appropriate method:

Research Approach	Method
Scientific	Community work
Naturalistic	Living lab
PAR	Ethnography
Pragmatic	Survey

6. Which approaches are researcher led, and which are user led?
7. Why is it important to maximise the involvement of people with dementia in research?
8. What are some of the risks associated with involving people with dementia in research?
9. What safeguards can be put in place to protect people with dementia when participating in research?
10. What can be done to enable people with dementia to participate more meaningfully?

REFERENCES

Alzheimer's Research Trust. 2010. *Dementia 2010: The Prevalence, Economic Cost and Research Funding of Dementia Compared with Other Major Diseases*. Cambridge, UK: Alzheimer's Research Trust.

Alzheimer's Society. 2007. *Dementia UK*. London: Alzheimer's Society.

Alzheimer's Society. 2012. *Dementia 2012: A National Challenge*. London: Alzheimer's Society.

Alzheimer's Society. 2013. *Dementia 2013: The Hidden Voice of Loneliness*. London: Alzheimer's Society.

Bartlett, R., & O'Connor, D. 2007. From personhood to citizenship: Broadening the lens for dementia practice and research. *Journal of Aging Studies*, 21(2): 107–118.

Bergvall-Kåreborn, B., & Ståhlbröst, A. (2010) Living lab: An open and user-centric design approach. In *Information and Communication Technologies, Society and Human Beings: Theory and Framework*, edited by Haftor, D., & Mirijamdotter, A., 190–207. London: IGI Global.

Budweg, S., Schaffers, H., Ruland, R., Kristensen, K., & Prinz, W. 2015. Enhancing collaboration in communities of professionals using a living lab approach. *Production Planning & Control*, 22(5–6): 594–609.

Crooks, V.C., Lubben, J., Petitti, D.B., Little, D., & Chiu, V. 2008. Social network, cognitive function, and dementia incidence among elderly women. *American Journal of Public Health*, 98(7): 1221–1227.

Department for Constitutional Affairs. 2007. *Mental Capacity Act 2005 Code of Practice*. London: The Stationary Office.

Department of Health. 2009. *Living Well with Dementia: A National Dementia Strategy*. London: Department of Health.

Department of Health. 2013. *The Prime Minister's Challenge on Dementia: Delivering Major Improvements in Dementia Care and Research by 2015: Annual Report of Progress*. London: Department of Health.

Department of Health. 2015. *Prime Minister's challenge on dementia 2020*. London: Department of Health.

Eckhardt, E., & Anastas, J. 2007. Research methods with disabled populations. *Journal of Social Work in Disability & Rehabilitation*, 6(1–2): 233–249.

Ericsson, I., Hellström, I., & Kjellström, S. 2011. Sliding interactions: An ethnography about how persons with dementia interact in housing with care for the elderly. *Dementia*, 10: 523–538.

Fals-Borda, O. 1997. Participatory action research in Colombia: Some personal feelings. In *Participatory Action Research: International Contexts and Consequences*, edited by McTaggart, R., 107–120. Albany NY: State University of New York Press.

Finfgeld-Connett, D. 2008. Concept synthesis of the art of nursing. *Journal of Advanced Nursing*, 62(3): 381–388.

Fratiglioni, L., Wang, H.X., Ericsson, K., Maytan, M., & Winblad, B. 2000. The influence of social network on the occurrence of dementia: A community-based longitudinal study. *Lancet*, 355: 1315–1319.

Greenhalgh, T., & Wieringa, S. 2011. Is it time to drop the 'knowledge translation' metaphor? A critical literature review. *Journal of the Royal Society of Medicine*, 104: 501–509.

Hanley, B., Bradburn, J., Barnes, M., Evans, C., Goodare, H., Kelson, M., Kent, A., Oliver, S., Thomas, S., & Wallcraft, J. 2004. *Involving the Public in NHS, Public Health and Social Care Research: Briefing Notes for Researchers*. Eastleigh, UK: Involve.

Holwerda, T.J., Deeg, D.J.H., Beekman, A.T.F., van Tilburg, T.G., Stek, M.L., Jonker, C., & Schoevers, R.A. 2014. Feelings of loneliness, but not social isolation, predict dementia onset: Results from the Amsterdam Study of the Elderly (AMSTEL). *Journal of Neurology, Neurosurgery, and Psychiatry*, 85: 135–142.

Johnson, R.B., Onwuegbuzie, A.J., & Turner, L.A. 2007. Toward a definition of mixed methods research. *Journal of Mixed Methods Research*, 1(2): 112–133.

McKeown, J., Clarke, A., Ingleton, C., & Repper, J. 2010. Actively involving people with dementia in qualitative research. *Journal of Clinical Nursing*, 19: 1935–1943.

McLaughlin, H. 2010. Keeping service user involvement in research honest. *British Journal of Social Work*, 40, 1591–1608.

Moos, I., & Bjorn, A. 2006. Use of the life story in the institutional care of people with dementia: a review of intervention studies. *Ageing Society*, 26(3): 431–454.

Murray, A. 2013. The Mental Capacity Act and dementia research. *Nursing Older People*, 25(3): 14–20.

Nomura, M., Makimoto, K., Kato, M., Shiba, T., Matsuura, C., Shigenobu, K., Ishikawa, T., Matsumoto, N., & Ikeda, M. 2009. Empowering older people with early dementia and family caregivers: A participatory action research study. *International Journal of Nursing Studies*, 46: 431–441.

Petr, C.G., & Walter, U. 2009. Evidence-based practice: A critical reflection. *European Journal of Social Work*, 12(2): 221–232.

Proctor, G. 2001. Listening to older women with dementia: Relationships, voices and power. *Disability and Society*, 16(3): 361–376.

Reason, P. 2003. Pragmatist philosophy and action research: Readings and conversation with Richard Rorty. *Action Research*, 1(1): 103–123.

Reason, P., & Bradbury, H. (Editors). 2001. *Handbook of Action Research: Participative Inquiry and Practice*. London: Sage.

Sackett, D.L., Rosenberg, W.M.C., Gray, J.A.M., Haynes, R.B., & Richardson, W.S. 1996. Evidence based medicine: what it is and what it isn't. *British Medical Journal*, 312: 71–72.

Shankar, A., Hamer, M., McMunn, A., & Steptoe, A. 2013. Social isolation and loneliness: Relationships with cognitive function during 4 years of follow-up in the English longitudinal study of ageing. *Psychosomatic Medicine*, 75(2): 161–170.

Smith, G. 2012. Conclusion: Psychological interventions and the mental health nurse's future development. In *Psychological Interventions*, edited by Smith, G., 155–164. Maidenhead, UK: Open University Press.

Smith, G. 2014. *Mental Health Nursing at a Glance*. Chichester, UK: Wiley Blackwell.

Tanner, D. 2013. Co-research with older people with dementia: Experience and reflections. *Journal of Mental Health*, 21(3): 296–306.

Weber, M.E.A. 2011. *Customer Co-creation in Innovations: A Protocol for Innovating with End Users*. Eindhoven, the Netherlands: Eindhoven University of Technology.

Woods, L., Smith, G., Pendleton, J., & Parker, D. 2013. *Innovate Dementia Baseline Report: Shaping the Future for People Living with Dementia*. Liverpool, UK: Liverpool John Moores University.

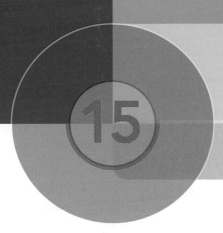

The way forward

GRAHAME SMITH

AIM

- To examine the future development of the practitioner working in dementia care

OBJECTIVES

- Consider the importance of clinical leadership as a component of expert practice
- Recognise the significance of learning from people living with dementia
- Identify the features of lifelong learning and its relationship to continuing professional development
- Describe expert practice
- Consider the role critical reflection has within learning from practice

OVERVIEW

Over recent years, there has been a significant focus on supporting staff in health and social care to develop the skills and knowledge to provide good quality dementia care (Higher Education for Dementia Network [HEDN], 2013; Department of Health [DH], 2009; Moyle et al., 2011). To develop the right skills and knowledge the practitioner needs not only to demonstrate the required level of competency but also to be an effective lifelong learner (HEDN, 2013; Smith, 2012a):

A number of frameworks have been developed which set out knowledge and skills requirements. … However these need supporting through effective training, education, continuous professional and vocational development in dementia. (HEDN, 2013: 3)

To ensure that the … nurse is adaptive to change and can also deliver high-quality care, the … nurse needs not only to have a full set of baseline skills but also continue to develop and enhance their skills as part of a lifelong learning journey. (Smith, 2012a: 157)

On this basis this chapter considers the skills and knowledge required to deliver high-quality dementia care and what the practitioner needs to do to be a lifelong learner. As a useful starting point the Curriculum for UK Dementia Education developed by HEDN (2013) describes formal development within dementia care as needing to be 'systematic, relevant, and meaningful'; it also has to encourage 'critical thinking and reflection'. In addition the practitioner has to be an effective leader and an effective change agent who is caring and compassionate (HEDN, 2013). Practitioners building on their formal education during their lifelong learning journey should underpin their practice with values (HEDN, 2013: 8) which enable people with dementia to

- Be empowered
- Exercise their rights and choices
- Maintain their identity
- Be treated with equity, dignity and respect
- Access an early and accurate diagnosis of dementia
- Maintain their best level of physical, mental, social and emotional well-being
- Maintain and expand their social and personal networks
- Be given information that they understand and enables their decision-making
- Access quality services with respect to their diverse needs
- Be as safe and independent as possible
- Expect a good and respectful death

To shape our journey through this chapter let us first consider the scenario that follows; this scenario is used in each section of the chapter to assist in the learning process:

Martha is a newly qualified mental health nurse who has just been employed as a staff nurse on a 15-bed dementia ward. Martha feels nervous and unsure of her learning needs; she feels prepared by her prequalifying training but knows there is more to be done.

LEADERSHIP

Education can only raise standards of care if it is part of a systematic approach to quality enhancement, embracing the development of leadership and changing organisational cultures. (HEDN, 2013: 4)

A practitioner may think that being a leader relates to being in a formal leadership role, but in reality this is not the case. Being a leader is part of being a responsible and accountable practitioner; for nurses this journey starts during their preregistration nurse training (Nursing and Midwifery Council [NMC], 2010, 2015; Smith, 2014). Leadership skills and knowledge that the nurse should be competent in at the point of registration include leading and coordinating care that is safe, personalised and responsive to need; managing self and others; being self-aware, including being professionally and legally accountable; working effectively across professional and agency boundaries; actively engaging in lifelong learning, reflection and the supervision of others and recognising the value of evidence in practice (NMC, 2010; Smith, 2014; Callaghan & Crawford, 2009).

The learning journey does not stop after registration. Nurses will further develop their generic skills; they also may develop skills and knowledge in a number of specialist areas or they may focus on one specialist area (Smith, 2012a). Concentrating on dementia, being a leader in the delivery of high-quality dementia care, will require the practitioner to be an expert in health promotion, assessment, communication, partnership working, inclusive practice, delivering person-centred care, evidence-based practice, understanding the ethical and legal context, and end of life care (HEDN, 2013). Benner (1982) made the following point about expertise and experience which is explored in further detail in the section on expert practice:

At the expert level, the performer no longer relies on an analytical principle (rule, guideline, maxim) to connect her/his understanding of the situation to an appropriate action. The expert nurse, with her/his enormous background of experience, has an intuitive grasp of the situation and zeros in on the accurate region of the problem without wasteful consideration of a large range of unfruitful possible problem situations. (Benner, 1982: 405)

Being an expert does not mean just possessing the requisite skills and knowledge; it also means understanding the nature of being an expert and how this relates to the leading and influencing of others (Morrison & Symes, 2011). Within the dementia field effective leadership is viewed as a key component in the drive to improve care quality (Francis, 2013; Moyle et al., 2011); to be effective, the nurse must also be emotionally intelligent in a way that engenders trust (Smith, 2014; Goleman, 1998). Let us return to Martha:

Martha starts her leadership journey by identifying her strengths and the areas she needs to develop through regularly engaging in clinical supervision. Martha has been assigned a preceptor and they have formulated an agreed plan of action. Part of this plan is for Martha to 'shadow' expert practitioners. During this process Martha has started to cultivate the following leadership qualities and traits she has identified in others: be authentic and motivated and have integrity; be an active listener; clearly communicate your intention; listen to others; be constructive; value quality; and be adaptable.

LEARNING FROM PEOPLE LIVING WITH DEMENTIA

Actively listening is an important part of being a leader and an expert. Being a skilled listener when working with people living with dementia provides the opportunity for the practitioner to really understand their needs and values (Smith, 2012b, 2012c). The challenge for the practitioner is that though working with people with dementia can be rewarding, it can also be stressful, and it is not unusual for practitioners to develop negative assumptions (Yamashita, Kinney, & Lokon, 2011; Allan & Killick, 2014; DH, 2009). These assumptions can be viewed as stemming from society's negative portrayal of dementia, using such terms for people with dementia as burden, suffering, and victim (Yamashita et al., 2011; Zeilig, 2014). Listening gives the practitioner the opportunity to really connect with the person with dementia, to put their assumptions aside and to be person centred and understand the person's real-life experiences, their hopes, aspirations, and values (Yamashita, Kinney, & Lokon, 2011; Mast, 2014; Smith, 2012b, 2012c).

It is important to recognise people living with dementia have the same wants and needs as everyone else—they want to be and feel in control; they want their life to be meaningful; they want to be empowered; and they want to feel of value to society (Yamashita, Kinney, & Lokon, 2011; Mast, 2014; Moyle et al., 2011). Due to the communication challenges some people with dementia face the practitioner has to be flexible and adaptive in the way he or she manages the communication process and be open and receptive to different forms of communication, especially where people with dementia have difficulty in expressing themselves verbally (Yamashita, Kinney, & Lokon, 2011; Smith, 2014). Building on the effective use of communication skills, a practitioner can then look to establish a therapeutic relationship which is collaborative and provides a robust platform from which to deliver a number of psychological interventions (Smith, 2012b, 2014). The importance of the therapeutic relationship especially within a context should not be underestimated:

> The therapeutic relationship within the mental health field, unlike most health-care relationships, tends to be both the medium for treatment as well as, in most cases, the main treatment itself. (Smith, 2012b: 4)

The expert practitioner will recognise that working with people with dementia has now moved away from just focusing on symptom control to focusing more on improving their quality of life and well-being (Woods et al., 2013; Kitwood, 1997; DH, 2009; Moyle et al., 2011). Returning to Martha:

Martha's plan of action also includes identifying the types of psychological interventions for which she will need to be proficient to enable her to learn from people with dementia:

- Establishing a therapeutic relationship based on a person centred approach
- Providing tailored support that focuses on assisting the individual to meet his or her physical needs
- Working on improving cognitive ability, including memory
- Reducing disorientation through memory prompts, both verbal and environmental
- Being empathetic to the emotional context and meanings of someone experiencing memory loss and confusion
- Providing behavioural strategies that positively modify challenging behaviour (Smith, 2014: 51)

LIFELONG LEARNING

Within the health and social care arena, the notions of continuing professional development (CPD) and lifelong learning have become synonymous. In the next section we explore CPD in greater depth. At this stage it is sufficient to say that lifelong learning has a broader context which encompasses CPD (Smith, 2012b). Lifelong learning is mentioned often, though it has no generally accepted definition. For the purposes of this section lifelong learning is viewed as a

… holistic process of developing skills and understanding (Sharples, 2000; Tuijnman & Bostrom, 2002; NMC, 2008; Fox, 2009; Kedge and Appleby, 2009). The process is also viewed as learning across the lifespan of an individual and it includes learning outside such formal settings as educational institutions and programmes (Tuijnman and Bostrom, 2002). (Smith, 2012a: 158)

The idea of lifelong learning being a holistic process is important in that it means learning is not confined only to the workplace or to a formal period of study (Smith, 2012a; Tuijnman & Bostrom, 2002; Kedge & Appleby, 2009; Fox, 2009). The implication is that the learner determines learning, and it can have value regardless of the setting or where it occurred in the person's life span (Smith, 2012a; Tuijnman & Bostrom, 2002; Blaschke, 2012). This broad view of lifelong learning having value needs to have a reflective component in which experiences are actively reflected on and learning is identified, explored, and appreciated (Smith, 2012a; Blaschke, 2012). According to Blaschke (2012), lifelong learners or 'capable people' demonstrate the following:

- Self-efficacy: Knowing how to learn and continuously reflect on the learning process
- Communication and teamwork skills: Working well with others and being openly communicative
- Creativity: Applying competencies to new and unfamiliar situations and by being adaptable and flexible in approach
- Positive values (Blaschke, 2012: 59)

Lifelong learning and being an expert practitioner are interdependent. On a regular basis expert practitioners have to deal with complex situations for which the outcome is not always certain. To deal with this uncertainty, they have to utilise learning which may or may not have occurred within a practice setting (Franks, 2004; Smith, 2012a; Finfgeld-Connett, 2008; Blaschke, 2012). The expert practitioners will then learn from these situations by reflecting in a rational, logical, and emotionally intelligent way, the outcome being that they will continuously seek to improve their practice (Smith, 2012a; Eason, 2010). Let us return to Martha:

Martha, who is meeting regularly with her preceptor, is being encouraged to think about her learning within a wider context. This includes recognising that

- Reflection as a core component of the lifelong-learning journey takes time to get right.
- Other life skills and knowledge can be valuable within the practice setting.
- Drive and commitment to continually develop are important.
- The preceptorship process is a step in the journey towards expert practice.

CONTINUING PROFESSIONAL DEVELOPMENT

Continuing professional development is a narrow view of lifelong learning albeit an important view. Professionally health and social field practitioners have to maintain their registration and are expected to engage in CPD (NMC, 2011; Health and Care Professions Council [HCPC], 2012). Regulatory bodies in this field set CPD standards to which the practitioner has to adhere.

For nursing these standards are the NMC's postregistration education and practice (Prep) standards. These standards are currently under review (Kedge & Appleby, 2009; NMC, 2011). Their role is to 'ensure that nurses and midwives keep their skills and knowledge up to date and maintain and develop their competence' (NMC, 2015: 17). Prep does this by providing a framework that aims to 'encourage the nurse to think and reflect and it assists the nurse to demonstrate that they are keeping up to date and developing their practice' (NMC, 2011: 2). There are two separate Prep standards which affect a nurse's registration (NMC, 2011): the Prep (practice) standard and the Prep (CPD) standard.

The Prep (CPD) standard (NMC, 2011: 8) requires the nurse to

1. Undertake at least 35 hours of learning activity relevant to your practice during the three years prior to your renewal of registration
2. Maintain a personal professional profile of your learning activity
3. Comply with any request from the NMC to audit how you have met these requirements.

In addition the NMC (2011) Prep (practice) requirement states:

In order to meet the practice standard you must have undertaken the 450 hours in your capacity as a nurse or midwife. (NMC, 2011: 4)

Not all registered practitioners working in the dementia field are nurses. On this basis it is useful to take a look at the HCPC (2012) position:

You must undertake CPD to stay registered with us. We have set standards which your CPD must meet. (HCPC, 2012: 2)

The HCPC's standards for CPD are:

1. Maintain a continuous, up-to-date and accurate record of their CPD activities;
2. Demonstrate that their CPD activities are a mixture of learning activities relevant to current or future practice;
3. Seek to ensure that their CPD has contributed to the quality of their practice and service delivery;
4. Seek to ensure that their CPD benefits the service user; and
5. Upon request, present a written profile (which must be their own work and supported by evidence) explaining how they have met the standards for CPD. (HCPC, 2012: 6)

Returning to Martha, let us look at how this professional requirement for nurses fits within Martha's lifelong learning journey:

Martha recognises that to provide evidence she meets the Prep standards she will need to keep a portfolio. Martha decides to use the following approach to help her write and organise her portfolio (Timmins & Duffy, 2011):

- She committed to actively engage in the process of writing her portfolio.
- The portfolio organisation clearly articulated Martha's learning journey (dated throughout).

- Local and national proficiencies were used as part of a structure, with each proficiency linking to a plan of action and a progress section.
- Her reflective endeavours (preceptorship process) were captured within her portfolio, including what she had learnt and what she needed to do to improve her practice.
- Martha referenced her learning to both the professional requirements for Prep and the NMC's code of conduct.
- Any underpinning evidence base was also clearly referenced.

EXPERT PRACTICE

Trying to define expert practice is similar to trying to define lifelong learning; Jasper (1994), in a nursing context, took the following view:

> Although the term 'expert' is used commonly in nursing practice and the nursing literature, it is apparent from this analysis and subsequent discussion that the term is ambiguous and difficult to clarify. The attribution of expertise remains linked to subjective criteria and reputation, with all of the defining attributes (knowledge, experience, pattern recognition and recognition by others) having loosely defined parameters. (Jasper, 1994: 775)

Even though there is not a clear and agreed definition of expert practice, there are a number of competency frameworks in use in the dementia field which use the terms expert and/or expert practice (Traynor, Inoue, & Crookes, 2011). The use of these terms in nursing is heavily influenced by the seminal work of Patricia Benner who proposed the following description of the expert nurse's learning journey:

1. Novice: Learning to be a nurse
2. Advanced Beginner: Starting to contextualise theories via practical experience
3. Competent: Can manage most standard clinical situations but lacks speed and flexibility
4. Proficient: Looks at situations holistically, can recognise non-standard situations
5. Expert: Not just reliant on rules to manage situation can also use tacit knowledge (Benner, 1982: 403–406)

Traynor, Inoue, and Crookes (2011) after reviewing a number of competency frameworks suggest that a competency framework for practitioners who work with people living with dementia should include the following:

- Understanding Dementia
- Recognising Dementia
- Effective Communication
- Assisting with Daily Living Activities
- Promoting a Positive Environment
- Ethical and Person-Centred Care
- Therapeutic Work
- Responding to the needs of Family Carers
- Preventative Work and Health Promotion
- Special Needs Groups (Traynor, Inoue, & Crookes, 2011: 1955)

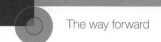

In addition, Traynor, Inoue, and Crookes (2011) proposed that these 'sets of competencies' should be evaluated using Benner's (1982) levels of expertise: novice, beginner, competent, proficient, and expert. Taking this view into consideration let us relate this to Martha:

Martha has decided that she would like to be expert in identification and assessment of dementia. To be competent Martha would be expected to be able to

- Recognise the signs and symptoms that would indicate the need for further assessment
- Articulate the assessment and diagnostic process
- Describe interventions that may be helpful in given situations
- Map the support networks available in a given area
- Develop an innovative toolkit for assertive outreach and crisis intervention (HEDN, 2013: 24–25)

Using Benner's (1982) framework as a template, Martha recognises she is competent in

- Recognising the signs and symptoms that would indicate the need for further assessment
- Articulating the assessment and diagnostic process
- Describing interventions that may be helpful in given situations
- Mapping the support networks available in a given area and is developing competency in
- Developing an innovative toolkit for assertive outreach and crisis intervention

Martha's competency stems from her professional training as a mental health nurse, for which Martha has developed a prescribed set of skills and knowledge (NMC, 2010; Smith, 2012b). On qualifying, Martha has further developed these generic mental health nursing skills and knowledge in a dementia care context through her experiences as a practitioner (Smith, 2012b; Higgins, Spencer, & Kane, 2010; Lyneham, Parkinson, & Denholm, 2008). At this stage in her development, Martha acknowledges that to support her on her journey towards being an expert in the dementia care field, she will need to undertake a programme of study that is dementia specific (HEDN, 2013). A challenge for Martha is knowing when she has arrived at the level of an expert. The following may help:

Both expert and newly qualified mental health nurses will be able to cope with a range of situations, but where the newly qualified nurse will lack some 'speed and flexibility' the expert nurse is not only more 'analytical and fluid' but they can also recognise and skilfully deal with an unexpected clinical situation. (Smith, 2012a: 160)

CRITICAL REFLECTION

Reflection is an integral part of expert practice; being skilled in critical reflection facilitates the expert practitioner to learn from his or her practice experiences (Morrison & Symes, 2011; Finfgeld-Connett, 2008; Jasper & Rolfe, 2011). Though practice experiences can be generalised, in essence, like all experiences, they are unique to the individual. Therefore any subsequent learning will also have a unique and personal element (Finfgeld-Connett, 2008; Smith, 2012a). This does not mean that reflection does not have a general or common structure; it just means that the experience that is processed by the practitioner will be personal to them. Generally the process of reflection will require the practitioner to reexamine a particular practice experience with a focus on changing their practice for the better (Smith, 2012a). Structurally it will have the following common elements:

- Identifying and describing the experience/s
- Examining the experience in depth, teasing out the key issues, what did I think at the time, how did I feel?
- Processing the issues, how do the issues relate to practice, what have I learnt?
- In the light of examining this experience, what actions do I need to take, how can I improve my practice? (Smith, 2014: 85)

The first stage of reflection, and sometimes the hardest stage, requires the practitioner to identify a critical incident that arose from their practice; in other words the practitioner needs to systematically examine their practice (Freshwater, 2011; Crowe & O'Malley, 2006; Gould & Masters, 2004; Crowe & O'Malley, 2006; Brimblecombe et al., 2007). One way of doing this is to actively engage in the process of clinical supervision: 'a protected period time where a practitioner is facilitated to reflect on their practice' (Bond & Holland, 2011: 15). A number of clinical supervision models are available, though on a professional level, whatever model is used, the nurse should ensure the process

- Supports practice and enables the practitioner to maintain and promote standards of care
- Facilitates a practice-focused professional relationship involving a practitioner reflecting on practice guided by a skilled supervisor
- Is developed by practitioners and managers according to local circumstances; ground rules should be agreed so that practitioners and supervisors approach clinical supervision openly, confidently and are aware of what is involved
- Ensures all practitioners have access to clinical supervision and each supervisor should supervise a realistic number of practitioners
- Confirms supervisors are adequately prepared with the principles and relevance of clinical supervision being included in pre- and post-registration education programmes
- Ensures that the practice of clinical supervision is evaluated locally with a focus on evaluating how it influences care, practice standards and the service (Smith, 2014: 85)

Returning to Martha:

Martha is struggling to critically reflect on her clinical experiences and on this basis Martha's clinical supervisor suggests Martha use the following questions to assist in her reflective endeavours (Crowe & O'Malley, 2006; Smith, 2012a):

- What is the issue and what is concerning about it?
- What justifications are provided for the current state of affairs?
- What are the social, cultural, political and historical factors that underpin and maintain this current state of affairs?
- How does the practice/situation impact on the service user?

- What options are available to do things differently?
- How will you justify doing things differently?
- What does the research or evidence base say about doing things differently?

CHAPTER SUMMARY

Actively listening is an important key part of being an expert practitioner; it affords an opportunity for the practitioner to really understand the needs and values of people living with dementia.

Practitioners in the dementia care field need to have the right skills and knowledge. They also need to be committed lifelong learners. Lifelong learning is a broad concept which encompasses CPD; it is also difficult to define. CPD is a narrow view of lifelong learning, albeit a very important view; regulatory bodies in this field set CPD standards to which the practitioner has to adhere.

Being a clinical leader is not necessarily fixed to a formal role. It is part of being a clinical practitioner.

There is no clear and agreed definition of expert practice though there are a number of competency frameworks in use in the dementia field which use the term *expert practice*. The use of this term in nursing is heavily influenced by the seminal work of Patricia Benner.

Reflection is an integral part of expert practice; being skilled in critical reflection facilitates the expert practitioner to learn from their practice experiences.

REFLECTION ON LEARNING

1. List the HEDN (2013) values which enable people with dementia.
2. What can clinical leadership change?
3. Active listening is a part of what?
4. Why do practitioners in the dementia care field have to be open and receptive to different forms of communication?
5. Define lifelong learning.
6. What do lifelong learners (capable people) demonstrate?
7. Describe the NMC's (2011) standards for CPD.
8. Describe the HCPC's (2012) standards for CPD.
9. Describe Benner's (1982) features of expert practice.
10. What are the common elements of structured reflection?

REFERENCES

Allan, K., & Killick, J. 2014. Communication and relationships: An inclusive social world. In *Excellence in Dementia Care: Research into Practice*, 2nd Edition, edited by Downs, M., & Bowers, B., 240–255. Maidenhead, UK: Open University Press.

Benner, P. 1982. From novice to expert. *The American Journal of Nursing*, 82(3), 402–407.

Blaschke, L.M. 2012. Heutagogy and lifelong learning: A review of heutagogical practice and self-determined learning. *International Review of Research in Open & Distance Learning*, 13(1): 56–71.

Bond, M., & Holland, S. 2011. *Skills of Clinical Supervision for Nurses: A Practical Guide for Supervisees, Clinical Supervisors and Managers: Supervision in Context*, 2nd edition. Maidenhead, UK: Open University Press.

Brimblecombe, N., Tingle, A., Tunmore, R., & Murrell, T. 2007. Implementing holistic practices in mental health nursing: A national consultation. *International Journal of Nursing Studies*, 44: 339–348.

Callaghan, P., & Crawford, P. 2009. Evidence-based mental health nursing practice. In *Mental Health Nursing Skills*, edited by Callaghan, P., Playle, J., & Cooper, L., 33–43. Oxford, UK: Oxford University Press.

Crowe, M.T., & O'Malley, J. 2006. Teaching critical reflection skills for advanced mental health nursing practice: a deconstructive–reconstructive approach. *Journal of Advanced Nursing*, 56(1): 79–87.

Department of Health. 2009. *Living Well with Dementia: A National Dementia Strategy*. London: Department of Health.

Eason, T. 2010. Lifelong learning: Fostering a culture of curiosity. *Creative Nursing*, 16(4): 155–159.

Finfgeld-Connett, D. 2008. Concept synthesis of the art of nursing. *Journal of Advanced Nursing*, 62(3): 381–388.

Francis, R. 2013. *Report of the Mid Staffordshire NHS Foundation Trust Public Inquiry— Executive Summary*. London: Stationery Office.

Franks, V. 2004. Evidence-based uncertainty in mental health nursing. *Journal of Psychiatric and Mental Health Nursing*, 11: 99–105.

Freshwater, M. 2011. Clinical supervision and reflective practice. In *Critical Reflection in Practice: Generating Knowledge for Care*, 2nd edition, edited by Rolfe, G., Jasper, M., & Freshwater, D., 100–126. Basingstoke, UK: Palgrave Macmillan.

Goleman, D. 1998. What makes a leader? In *Creative Management Development*, 3rd edition, edited by Henry, J., 120–132. London: Sage.

Gould, B., & Masters, H. 2004. Learning to make sense: The use of critical incident analysis in facilitated reflective groups of mental health student nurses. *Learning in Health and Social Care*, 3(2): 53–63.

Health and Care Professions Council. 2012. *Information for registrants: Continuing professional development and your registration*. London: Heath & Care Professions Council.

Higgins, G., Spencer, R.L., & Kane, R. 2010. A systematic review of the experiences and perceptions of the newly qualified nurse in the United Kingdom. *Nurse Education Today*, 30: 499–508.

Higher Education for Dementia Network. 2013. *A Curriculum for UK Dementia Education*. London: Dementia UK.

Jasper, M. 1994. Expert: A discussion of the implications of the concept as used in nursing. *Journal of Advanced Nursing*, 20: 769–776.

Jasper, M., & Rolfe, G. 2011. Critical reflection and the emergence of professional knowledge. In *Critical Reflection in Practice: Generating Knowledge for Care*, 2nd edition, edited by Rolfe, G., Jasper, M., & Freshwater, D., 1–10. Basingstoke, UK: Palgrave Macmillan.

Kedge, S., & Appleby, B. 2009. Promoting a culture of curiosity within nursing practice. *British Journal of Nursing*, 18(10): 635–637.

Kitwood, T. 1997. *Dementia Reconsidered*. London: Open University Press.

Lyneham, J., Parkinson, C., & Denholm, C. 2008. Explicating Benner's concept of expert practice: Intuition in emergency nursing. *Journal of Advanced Nursing*, 64(4): 380–387.

Mast, B. 2014. Whole person assessment and care planning. In *Excellence in Dementia Care: Research into Practice*, 2nd edition, edited by Downs, M., & Bowers, B., 290–302. Maidenhead, UK: Open University Press.

Morrison, S.M., & Symes, L. 2011. An integrative review of expert nursing practice. *Journal of Nursing Scholarship*, 43(2): 163–170.

Moyle, W., Venturto, L., Griffiths, S., Grimbeekc, P., McAllister, M., Oxlade, D., & Murfield, J. 2011. Factors influencing quality of life for people with dementia: A qualitative perspective. *Aging & Mental Health*, 15(8): 970–977.

Nursing and Midwifery Council. 2010. *Standards for Pre-registration Nursing Education*. London: Nursing and Midwifery Council.

Nursing and Midwifery Council. 2011. *The Prep Handbook*. London: Nursing and Midwifery Council.

Nursing and Midwifery Council. 2015. *The Code: Professional Standards of Practice and Behaviour for Nurses and Midwives*. London: Nursing and Midwifery Council.

Owen, S., & Fox, C. 2009. Personal and professional development. In *Mental Health Nursing Skills*, edited by Callaghan, P., Playle, J., & Cooper, L., 223–231. Oxford, UK: Oxford University Press.

Sharples, M. 2000. The design of personal mobile technologies for lifelong learning. *Computers & Education*, 34: 177–193.

Smith, G. 2012a. Conclusion: Psychological interventions and the mental health nurse's future development. In *Psychological Interventions*, edited by Smith, G., 155–164. Maidenhead, UK: Open University Press.

Smith, G. 2012b. An introduction to psychological interventions. In *Psychological Interventions*, edited by Smith, G., 1–10. Maidenhead, UK: Open University Press.

Smith, G. 2012c. Psychological interventions within an ethical context. In *Psychological Interventions*, edited by Smith, G., 143–154. Maidenhead, UK: Open University Press.

Smith, G. 2014. *Mental Health Nursing at a Glance*. Chichester, UK: Wiley Blackwell.

Timmins, F., & Duffy, A. 2011. *Writing Your Nursing Portfolio: A Step-by-Step Guide*. Maidenhead, UK: Open University Press.

Traynor, V., Inoue, K., & Crookes, P. 2011. Literature review: Understanding nursing competence in dementia care. *Journal of Clinical Nursing*, 20(13–14): 1948–1960.

Tuijnman, A., & Bostrom, A. 2002. Changing notions of lifelong education and lifelong learning. *International Review of Education*, 48(1/2): 93–110.

Woods, L., Smith, G., Pendleton, J., & Parker, D. 2013. *Innovate Dementia Baseline Report: Shaping the Future for People Living with Dementia*. Liverpool, UK: Liverpool John Moores University.

Yamashita, T., Kinney, J.M., & Lokon, E.J. 2011. The impact of a gerontology course and a service-learning program on college students' attitudes toward people with dementia. *Journal of Applied Gerontology*, 32(2): 139–163.

Zeilig, H. 2014. Representations of people with dementia in the media and in literature. In *Excellence in Dementia Care: Research into Practice*, 2nd edition, edited by Downs, M., & Bowers, B., 78–90. Maidenhead, UK: Open University Press.

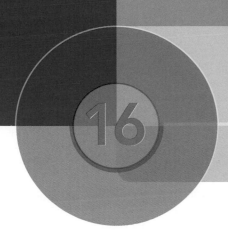

Conclusion

16

GRAHAME SMITH

SUMMARY

I hope you have found this book useful and while reading it you felt optimistic about how you can enable people living with dementia to live well (Department of Health [DH], 2009; Department of Health, Social Services and Public Safety [DHSSPS], 2011; Welsh Assembly Government, 2011; Scottish Government, 2013). It is recognised that the UK population is aging and as a potential consequence the number of people living with dementia will significantly increase. On the basis that the demand for dementia-related services will also increase, at the same time there is a societal move towards providing future services which are underpinned by assistive technology. The view is that services that use these technologies within an integrated approach will be more cost effective. Cost effective services are one strand in addressing this challenge. It is also vital that people living with dementia feel part of the wider community; in other words, society as a whole is dementia friendly. To be a dementia-friendly society, people living with dementia have to receive the right support at the right time.

Managing and potentially delaying the onset of dementia require multifaceted strategies which to be successful have to be based on a flexible approach, one that actively supports people with dementia living well. Part of living well is to have and maintain a healthy lifestyle. The health and social care practitioner as a health promoter has a role to play, which is to empower people living with dementia to make informed lifestyle choices. To be empowering, the practitioner has to have a good understanding of the condition; the practitioner has to be dementia aware. He or she also has to recognise that dementia can have general features, but each person will experience dementia in a unique way.

Individualised or person-centred care is an ethical and compassionate approach by which the practitioner draws on the skills and knowledge of people living with dementia as experts in their own care. Whatever the stage of the condition the practitioner has to have an appreciation of how dementia can impact on the caring process. Dementia as a condition and caring for someone with dementia can be stressful; negative attitudes can be a significant barrier to people with dementia living well with the condition. Practitioners can sometimes forget to really listen to people with dementia, so it is important to always

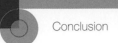

deliver care that is respectful and person centred and takes into account the value-laden nature of experiencing dementia. This approach should extend from early diagnosis to the end of life where care delivered has an emphasis on compassion and maintaining dignity.

To deliver person-centred care, the practitioner has to recognise that communication is a two-way process by which care is delivered in partnership through a therapeutic relationship as a 'doing with' rather than a 'doing to' approach. Possessing effective communication skills provides the practitioner with a good foundation on which to develop and deliver a range of different interventions. These interventions can be pharmacological or nonpharmacological; it is important that due to potential side effects medication is used carefully. In addition to the antidementia medications nonpharmacological approaches or psychological interventions are always preferable. A psychological intervention is a health and social care intervention which is underpinned by psychological methods and theory with the intention of improving biopsychosocial functioning. It is usually delivered through a therapeutically structured relationship. Psychological interventions for dementia include cognitive and behaviour-focused interventions. Psychological interventions can also reduce symptoms of depression and anxiety for people with dementia.

As the majority of people with dementia live at home, the practitioner has to be able to deliver care which helps people with dementia stay at home as long and as safely as possible. Preferably a person with dementia would age in place and be supported to live in his or her home setting until the end of life, however the need for residential care may be unavoidable due to the level of risk. To balance the need to safeguard and the need to promote independence the practitioner should utilise a risk enablement approach which focuses on a person's strengths rather than deficits. To be an effective enabler the practitioner must understand that people with dementia have rights and freedoms and these rights are protected by a number of legal frameworks. Irrespective of the care setting the environment has to be comforting, safe and understandable for people with dementia. Taking this into consideration the practitioner has to recognise that the environment as an intervention has a crucial role to play in the effective management of distressing symptoms in dementia.

Being strengths-focused also extends to the use of assistive technology; the practitioner must use these technologies to enable people living with dementia to live well. To do this the practitioner must know which technology to use; knowing should be based on having a true understanding of what it is like to live with dementia. This understanding is generated through supporting people living with dementia to talk about their everyday challenges, with a focus on the practitioner actively listening and then facilitating the journey towards discovering potential solutions. This journey should be underpinned by the relevant research base which should include approaches that are both 'top-down' researcher led and 'bottom-up' user led.

To really understand the needs and values of people living with dementia the practitioner has to be an active and skilled listener. To have the right skills and knowledge the practitioner has to be a committed lifelong learner who continually updates his or her knowledge and skills through a process of continuing professional development (CPD). Lifelong learning is a broad concept which encompasses CPD. It is difficult to define, however it can be structured through a number of competency frameworks in use within the dementia field. A key part of the lifelong journey for the practitioner is to engage with and be skilled in critical reflection, a process which enables the practitioner to learn from practice experiences.

REVISITING THE THEMES OF THE BOOK

As highlighted in the introduction to the book dementia is a personal and a societal challenge. Living with dementia can sometimes be overwhelming, though with the right support living well with dementia can become a reality rather than just an aspiration (Alzheimer's Society, 2014; DH, 2015). The practitioner's role is to meet this challenge with hope and compassion and being respectful even when dealing with the most challenging of behaviours (Francis, 2013; Hirst, Lane, & Stares, 2013). Delivering good quality care should be a given where the whole person is considered including the needs of their carers (DH, 2009; Kitwood, 1997).

It is accepted that to be expert the practitioner will need to access further learning, both informal and formal (Higher Education for Dementia Network [HEDN], 2013; Smith, 2012a). This book will in part help by signposting the practitioner to the relevant policies, strategies, and to the relevant research evidence. This approach will only work if the practitioner combines this with listening to, reflecting on, and valuing the voices of people living with dementia (Smith, 2012a).

Valuing also has to do with recognising strengths rather than just focusing on deficits. This can be difficult, especially where health and social care services have a tendency to be controlling and risk averse (DH, 2010; Rylance & Simpson, 2012; Smith, 2012c). Admittedly there are times when people with dementia can exhibit 'risky' behaviours and there may be a need to control, but this must be balanced against the need to enable (DH, 2010).

Enabling also creates a notional space where people living with dementia can be themselves and in some cases find their true potential. In Chapter 7, Tommy talks about feeling a sense of hopelessness after receiving a dementia diagnosis, and that carers are not always adequately supported. At the end of his narrative he highlights that through the right support he is living well and through his efforts and the efforts of others is being listened to. Carol, as a carer, talks about trying to normalise Terry's situation with a focus on seeing the person and all that makes them a person: the emotion, their memories, and a life lived together.

Listening to and learning from the narratives of people living with dementia are important; using other ways of doing this can also be equally important. Zeilig (2014) makes the point:

Poetry works in that space (in which we all operate) that is beyond the concrete world. It appeals to our remarkable ability to hold the known world in our heads when it is not in fact there: to imagine. If we can begin to imagine dementia we can also start to confront some of the assumptions that we have about this disease and its sufferers. Through its appeal to our imaginations and empathy, poetry brings into focus those slant truths that lie to the side of our vision. As the poet, Don Paterson, recently pointed out, 'If language could offer a full description of our experience, we wouldn't need poetry. Poetry is just language's self-corrective function, kicking in when the human encounters an otherness it can't properly articulate by the usual means' (Paterson, 2010: 83). Poetry helps us to configure the extreme otherness that is dementia. Poets use a heightened form of language (through metaphor, simile, metonymy, rhyme, rhythm and a host of other techniques) to try and capture the nature and experiences of this disease. (Zeilig, 2014: 172)

FINAL THOUGHTS

In the *Prime Minister's Challenge on Dementia 2020*, there is an aspiration which should resonate with all health and social care practitioners:

> By 2020 I want England to be: the best country in the world for dementia care and support and for people with dementia, their carers and families to live; and the best place in the world to undertake research into dementia and other neurodegenerative diseases. (DH, 2015: 2)

It does say England and the UK is wider than England; even so I believe this aspiration has value across all of the UK.

REFERENCES

Alzheimer's Society. 2014. *Dementia 2014: Opportunity for Change*. London: Alzheimer's Society.

Department of Health. 2009. *Living Well with Dementia: A National Dementia Strategy*. London: Department of Health.

Department of Health. 2010. *Nothing Ventured, Nothing Gained: Risk Guidance for People with Dementia*. London: Department of Health.

Department of Health. 2015. *Prime Minister's Challenge on Dementia 2020*. London: Department of Health.

Department of Health, Social Services and Public Safety. 2011. *Improving Dementia Services in Northern Ireland: A Regional Strategy*. Belfast: DHSSPS.

Edward, C. (Ed.). 2000. *Concise Routledge Encyclopaedia of Philosophy*. London: Routledge.

Francis, R. 2013. *Report of the Mid Staffordshire NHS Foundation Trust Public Inquiry—Executive Summary*. London: Stationery Office.

Higher Education for Dementia Network. 2013. *A Curriculum for UK Dementia Education*. London: Dementia UK.

Hirst, S.P., Lane, A., & Stares, R. 2013. Health promotion with older adults experiencing mental health challenges: A literature review of strength-based approaches. *Clinical Gerontologist*, 36(4): 329–355.

Kitwood, T. 1997. *Dementia Reconsidered*. London: Open University Press.

Paterson, D. 2010. The domain of the poem. *Poetry Review*, 100(4): 81–100.

Rylance, R., & Simpson, P. 2012. Psychological interventions and managing risk. In *Psychological Interventions in Mental Health Nursing*, edited by Smith, G., 11–23. Maidenhead, UK: Open University Press.

Scottish Government. 2013. *Scotland's National Dementia Strategy: 2013–2016*. Edinburgh: Scottish Government.

Smith, G. (2012a) Conclusion: Psychological interventions and the mental health nurse's future development. In *Psychological Interventions*, edited by Smith, G., 155–164. Maidenhead, UK: Open University Press.

Smith, G. 2012b. An introduction to psychological interventions. In *Psychological Interventions in Mental Health Nursing*, edited by Smith, G., 1–10. Maidenhead, UK: Open University Press.

Smith, G. 2012c. Psychological interventions within an ethical context. In *Psychological Interventions*, edited by Smith, G., 143–154. Maidenhead, UK: Open University Press.

Welsh Assembly Government. 2011. *National Dementia Vision for Wales*. Cardiff, Wales: Welsh Assembly Government.

Zeilig, H. 2014. Gaps and spaces: Representations of dementia in contemporary British poetry. *Dementia*, 13(2): 160–175.

Index